The Clinical Manual

D0096428

The Clinical Manual

JOHN BRADLEY
BMed Sci, DM, MRCP
Senior Registrar, Addenbrooke's Hospital,
Cambridge

DAVID RUBENSTEIN
MA, MD, FRCP
Physician, Addenbrooke's Hospital,
Cambridge

DAVID WAYNE
BM, MA, FRCP
Physician, James Paget
District General Hospital,
Gorleston, Great Yarmouth

OXFORD

Blackwell Scientific Publications

LONDON EDINBURGH BOSTON
MELBOURNE PARIS BERLIN VIENNA

© 1994 by
Blackwell Scientific Publications
Editorial Offices:
Osney Mead, Oxford OX2 0EL
25 John Street, London WC1N 2BL
23 Ainslie Place, Edinburgh
  EH3 6AJ
238 Main Street, Cambridge
  Massachusetts 02142, USA
54 University Street, Carlton
  Victoria 3053, Australia

Other Editorial Offices:
Librairie Arnette SA
1, rue de Lille
75007 Paris
France

Blackwell Wissenschafts-Verlag
  GmbH
Düsseldorfer Str. 38
D-10707 Berlin
Germany

Blackwell MZV
Feldgasse 13
A-1238 Wien
Austria

First published 1994

Set by Setrite Typesetters,
Hong Kong
Printed and bound in Great Britain
at the Alden Press Limited,
Oxford and Northampton

DISTRIBUTORS

Marston Book Services Ltd
PO Box 87
Oxford OX2 0DT
(Orders: Tel: 0865 791155
        Fax: 0865 791927
        Telex: 837515)

USA
Blackwell Scientific
  Publications, Inc.
238 Main Street
Cambridge, MA 02142
(Orders: Tel: 800 759-6102
        617 876-7000)

Canada
Times Mirror Professional
  Publishing, Ltd
130 Flaska Drive
Markham, Ontario L6G 1B8
(Orders: Tel: 800 268-4178
        416 470-6739)

Australia
Blackwell Scientific Publications
  Pty Ltd
54 University Street
Carlton, Victoria 3053
(Orders: Tel: 03 347-5552)

A catalogue record for this title
is available from the British Library

ISBN 0-632-03312-6 (BSP)
     0-86542-810-7 (4 Dragons)

Library of Congress
Cataloging in Publication Data

Bradley, John.
    The clinical manual/
    John Bradley, David
    Rubenstein, David Wayne.
      p.   cm.
    Includes bibliographical
    references and index.
    ISBN 0-632-03312-6
    1. Internal medicine —
Handbooks, manuals, etc.
I. Wayne, David. II. Title.
    [DNLM: 1. Clinical Medicine —
handbooks. WB 39 B811c 1994]
RC55.B73   1994
616 — dc20

Contents

Preface

It is easy to forget the culture shock when moving from the solid ground of the preclinical course (where all is defined, understood and classifiable — or so they say!) to the vague diffuse world of clinical practice where there seem to be no obvious fixed points, and the student feels totally at sea and in the way.

Our book covers this period and beyond by:

- introducing history taking and examination technique;
- refreshing the parts other anatomists never reached;
- outlining the key symptoms, signs, investigation and management of common diseases;
- highlighting the management of acute diseases which can kill, and hence require urgent action;
- guiding students through laboratory testing, X-rays, electrocardiograms (ECGs) and invasive techniques.

The book should be carried in clinics and on the ward for rapid reference, and space has been included at the end of the book for students to make notes and record their own observations. In addition, it provides for more thorough reading away from the hustle and anxiety of wards and clinics.

The authors would like to thank the following medical students and teachers, from Cambridge, London, Oxford and Sheffield, for their useful comments and advice during the preparation of this manuscript: O. Behzadi, F. Bhatti, A. Donald, J. Dougherty, A. Gill, L. Hamilton, D. Hunter, K. Lankester, D. O'Riordan, M. Pitcher, W. Sherlock and J. Stockwell.

Abbreviations

a	atrial systole/contraction
ACE	angiotensin-converting enzyme
ACTH	adrenocorticotrophic hormone
ADH	antidiuretic hormone
AF	atrial fibrillation
AIDS	acquired immunodeficiency syndrome
ALT	alanine aminotransferase
ANCA	anti-neutrophil cytoplasm antibodies
AP	anteroposterior
APSA	anistreplase
APTT	activated partial thromboplastin time
ASD	atrial septal defect
AST	aspartate aminotransferase
ATN	acute tubular necrosis
AV	atrioventricular
AVF	augmented voltage F
AVL	augmented voltage L
AVR	augmented voltage R
AZT	azidothymidine
BCG	bacillus Calmette-Guérin
BP	blood pressure
BPH	benign prostatic hypertrophy
C6	complement component 6
CABG	coronary artery bypass graft
CD	cluster of differentiation
CH_{50}	volume of serum (source of complement) required to produce haemolysis of 50% of standard quantity of sensitized red cells
CHO	carbohydrate
CK	creatine kinase
CK-MB	creatine kinase is formed by dimerization of two polypeptide chains, denoted B and M, giving rise to three different isoenzymes. The predominant isoenzyme in skeletal muscle is

	MM, whereas in brain it is BB. Cardiac muscle contains both MM and MB
CMV	cytomegalovirus
CNS	central nervous system
CO_2	carbon dioxide
CPK	creatine phosphokinase
CPR	cardiopulmonary resuscitation
^{51}Cr	chromium-51
CREST	calcinosis, Raynaud's phenomenon, (o)esophageal involvement, sclerodactyly, telangiectasia
CRP	C-reactive protein
CSF	cerebrospinal fluid
CT	computed tomography
CVA	cerebrovascular accident
CVP	central venous pressure
CXR	chest X-ray
D&C	dilatation of cervix with endometrial curettage
DC	direct current
DIC	disseminated intravascular coagulation
DMSA	dimercaptosuccinate
DNA	deoxyribonucleic acid
DTPA	diethylenetriamine penta-acetic acid
DU	duodenal ulcer
DVT	deep venous/vein thrombosis
EB	Epstein−Barr
ECG	electrocardiogram
EDTA	ethylenediamine tetra-acetic acid
EEG	electroencephalogram
EMG	electromyography
ENT	ear−nose−throat
ESR	erythrocyte sedimentation rate
F	female
FBC	full blood count
FDP	fibrin degradation product
FEV_1	forced expiratory volume in 1 second
FOB	faecal occult blood
FVC	forced vital capacity

GFR	glomerular filtration rate
γGT	gamma-glutamyl transferase
G6PD	glucose-6-phosphate dehydrogenase
GTN	glyceryl trinitrate
GU	gastric ulcer
H$^+$	hydrogen ion
Hb	haemoglobin
HepBcAg	hepatitis B core antigen
HepBeAg	hepatitis B internal component antigen
HepBsAg	hepatitis B surface antigen
HIV	human immunodeficiency virus
HLA	human leucocyte antigen
HOCM	hypertrophic obstructive cardiomyopathy
HSV	herpes simplex virus
IgM	immunoglobulin M
IM	intramuscularly
INR	international normalized ratio
ITU	intensive therapy unit
IV	intravenously
IVC	inferior vena cava
IVU	intravenous urography
JVP	jugular venous pulse
KPTT	kaolin partial thromboplastin time
LA	left arm
LAP	leucocyte alkaline phosphatase
LDH	lactate dehydrogenase
LDL	low density lipoprotein
LFTs	liver function tests
LIF	left iliac fossa
LL	left leg
LP	lumbar puncture
LV	left ventricular
LVF	left ventricular failure
M	male
MAOI	monoamine oxidase inhibitor
M band	monoclonal immunoglobulin band
MCH	mean corpuscular haemoglobin
MCHC	mean corpuscular haemoglobin concentration

MCP	metacarpophalangeal
MCV	mean corpuscular volume
MHC	major histocompatibility
MMR	mumps, measles, rubella
MRC	Medical Research Council
MRI	magnetic resonance imaging
MSU	mid-stream urine
NSAIDs	non-steroidal anti-inflammatory drugs
OA	osteoarthritic
PA	posteroanterior
$PaCO_2$	partial pressure of arterial carbon dioxide
PaO_2	partial pressure of arterial oxygen
PCV	packed cell volume
PEFR	peak expiratory flow rate
PFR	peak flow rate
PIP	proximal interphalangeal
PND	paroxysmal nocturnal dyspnoea
PT	prothrombin time
PTH	parathyroid hormone
PUO	pyrexia of unknown origin
PUVA	oral psoralens and exposure to UVA light
QT_c	QT interval corrected for heart rate
RA	right arm
RBC	red blood cell
RDW	red cell distribution width
RL	right leg
RNA	ribonucleic acid
RSR	M-shaped QRS complex
RSV	respiratory syncytial virus
rt-PA	alteplase
RV	right ventricular
SA	sinoatrial
SBE	subacute bacterial endocarditis
SCC	squamous cell carcinoma
SLE	systemic lupus erythematosus
SOCRATES	site, onset, character, radiation, associations, timing, exacerbating and relieving factors, severity
SVC	superior vena cava

SVT	supraventricular tachycardia
TB	tuberculosis
^{99m}Tc	technetium-99m
t.d.s.	*ter die sumendum* (three times a day)
THREAD	tuberculosis, hypertension, rheumatic fever, epilepsy, asthma, anxiety and arthritis, diabetes and depression
TIA	transient ischaemic attack
TSH	thyroid-stimulating hormone
TURP	transurethral resection of prostate
UC	ulcerative colitis
UV	ultraviolet
UVA	ultraviolet A
v	ventricular systole/contraction
VF	ventricular fibrillation
VMA	vanilmandelic acid
VSD	ventricular septal defect
VT	ventricular tachycardia
WBC	white blood cell
WHO	World Health Organization

1 History

1

INTRODUCTION

Taking the history is the most valuable part of any consultation. It allows the doctor to establish a relationship with the patient and in the majority of cases suggests the diagnosis. This can then be confirmed by physical examination and investigation.

THE DOCTOR–PATIENT RELATIONSHIP

Although communication skills are acquired throughout life, the doctor–patient relationship is unique. It relies on mutual trust and honesty, and is crucial to understanding the patient's illness and planning their management.

Several key points should be remembered in order to put the patient at ease and to define their problems.

Put the patient at ease
- Greet the patient by name: 'Good morning, Mrs Brown';
- introduce yourself and explain that you are a medical student;
- shake the patient's hand, or if they are unwell rest your hand on theirs;
- ensure that the patient is comfortable.

Define the patient's problems

Questioning Ask open rather than leading questions, but be prepared to redirect the patient if they talk at length about matters unrelated to their problem by asking more specific, probing questions.

Listening Patients readily recognize whether they have a doctor's full attention. They are not impressed if they have to repeat information, or if it becomes apparent by your questioning that you have missed information.

Responding Encourage the patient whilst they are presenting the story, with nods and gestures. Be sympathetic to problems. Avoid appearing surprised or reproachful.

Explaining As a student you may not feel able to fully interpret the patient's symptoms. However, some explanation of how you feel the consultation has helped, and what you are planning (e.g. discussing the problems with the patient's doctor) should be provided.

NB: A final and probably unnecessary reminder — none of the authors considers himself a keen dresser but it remains important to *look the part*.

• Patients, particularly if they are unwell or apprehensive, will readily become disturbed if the doctor looks untidy or appears unsympathetic.

When taking the history first find out why the patient has come for medical attention. Start by asking the general questions given in History box 1 (below) to define the presenting problem and its duration.

History box 1
General questions to ask the patient first

Tell me what seems to be the problem?
How long have you been unwell?
When did the symptoms start?
Not What brought you here?

Ask the patient when and how it all started. Asking what they were doing at the time may help them to recall events. Then take the patient step by step through the evolution of their history, dating critical events — what has happened since? Encourage the patient to explain their experience in their own words, rather than allowing them to provide a label for their symptoms. For example, the term 'indigestion' may signify flatulence, abdominal discomfort, abdominal pain or chest pain — ask the patient to describe exactly what they feel.

By allowing a patient to talk, a detailed history will often emerge. If a history is not forthcoming it is usually clear which system is involved and specific questions can be asked (see pp. 6–7). Don't ask questions that suggest answers, that is, don't lead the patient.

PAIN

One of the commonest presenting symptoms is pain, and the questions that need to be asked are listed in History box 2 (below).

History box 2
Questions to ask about pain (SOCRATES)

Site	Where exactly is the pain?
Onset	When did the pain start?
	Did it start suddenly or gradually?
Character	Describe the pain — sharp? knife-like? gripping? vice-like? burning? crushing?
Radiation	Does the pain spread anywhere? — to the arm? jaw? groin?
Associations	Is the pain accompanied by any other features?
Timing	Does the pain vary in intensity during the day?
Exacerbating and relieving factors	Does anything make the pain better or worse?
Severity	How bad is the pain?
	Does the pain interfere with daily activities or with sleep?

Character

Descriptions in terms of imaginary causes that patients have rarely endured are common. Certain descriptions, however, are used consistently to describe specific pains. These include:

- the sharp, knife-like pain of pleurisy;
- the gripping, vice-like pain of myocardial infarction;
- the burning pain of oesophagitis.

Bear in mind that elderly patients may find it difficult to describe pain.

Radiation

Pain may radiate from its site of origin; for example, cardiac pain may radiate to the arm or the jaw, whereas the pain of renal colic may radiate to the groin.

Accompanying features

Features of sweating, nausea and breathlessness often accompany cardiac pain, whereas acid reflux into the mouth may accompany pain from the oesophagus or stomach.

Timing

The timing of the pain can be important — the headache of raised intracranial pressure and the joint stiffness of rheumatoid arthritis are both worse on getting up in the morning.

Exacerbating and relieving factors

Angina worsens on exertion (and sometimes in the cold, after large meals or with emotion) and is relieved by rest; oesophagitis is worse when bending over and is relieved by milk and antacids.

Severity

Although assessment of the severity of the pain will depend on the individual, some idea can be obtained by asking if the pain interferes with daily activities or with sleep.

SYSTEMATIC ENQUIRY

Once the main reason for the patient seeking medical attention has been established, you need to find out about his or her general health by asking the questions listed in History box 3 on pp. 6–7. The enquiry is systematic — according to the different body systems.

If the answer to any question listed in History box 3 is yes, find out more about the symptom by asking relevant supplementary questions, which are discussed and listed on the following pages (pp. 5–41).

Cardiovascular and respiratory symptoms

Cough (History box 4, p. 7)

Cough is the response to irritation of the respiratory tract.

Lying flat often aggravates coughing and increases any associated breathlessness (see orthopnoea, pp. 9–10). Coughing at night, particularly in children, often indicates asthma.

History box 3
Questions to ask patients about their general health

If the answer to any of these questions is 'yes' supplementary questions detailed on pp. 5–41 should follow

Cardiovascular and respiratory function
Do you have a cough?
Do you cough anything up?
Have you ever smoked? — if so what, how many, and for how long?
Do you get short of breath?
Do you wheeze?
Do you get palpitations?
Do you get any chest pain?
Do your ankles swell?

Gastrointestinal function
Has there been any change in your appetite?
Has there been any change in your weight?
Have you suffered from nausea or vomiting?
Has there been any change in the character or frequency of your bowel movements?
Has there been any change in the colour and consistency of your stools?
Have you had any bleeding? — while vomiting (haematemesis)? rectally?

Genitourinary function
How often do you pass urine?
Do you have pain or burning on passing urine?
Do you have pain in the small of the back (renal angles)?
Is there any blood in your urine (haematuria)?
Do you have any sexual problems?

Specific questions for men
Do you have any penile discharge or venereal infection?
Do you have difficulty starting to pass urine (hesitancy or urgency), maintaining the flow of urine (poor stream), or stopping the flow of urine (terminal dribbling)?

Specific questions for women
Do you have any vaginal discharge?
When did your periods start?
Are your periods irregular?
How often do your periods occur and for how long do they last?

Do you have heavy bleeding (menorrhagia) or do you pass clots during your period?
When did your periods stop (menopause)?
Have you had any bleeding since your periods stopped?
How many children have you had, and when did you have them?
Did you have any complications during any pregnancy?

Musculoskeletal function
Have you any weakness in your arms or legs?
Do you have any stiffness in your joints or spine?
Do you have pain in your joints or spine?

Neurological function
Do you have any headaches?
Have you had any blackouts?
Have you had any fits?
Have you had any dizziness (feeling of instability or rotation)?
Do you get ringing in your ears (tinnitus)?
Do you get abnormal sensations or tingling in your hands or feet (paraesthesia)?
Have you noticed changes to your sense of hearing, smell, taste, vision?
Have you had any incontinence of urine or stools?
Do you get depressed?
Do you get anxious?

History box 4
Questions to ask about a cough

When did the cough start?
What makes the cough worse?
What makes the cough better?
Is the cough worse during the day or at night?

Common causes of a cough

- Pharyngitis/tonsillitis;
- sinusitis (due to post-nasal drip, in which secretions from the paranasal sinuses drip into and irritate the upper airways);
- laryngitis;
- bronchitis;
- asthma.

Less common causes

- Pneumonia;
- bronchial carcinoma;
- laryngeal carcinoma.

History box 5
Questions to ask about sputum

How much sputum do you cough up each day? — is it a spoonful? an eggcupful? a teacupful?
What colour is the sputum?
Is the sputum bloodstained?
Is the sputum frothy?

Sputum (History box 5, above)

Sputum is composed of mucous secretions, usually from the lower respiratory tract.

The production of vast amounts of sputum usually indicates bronchiectasis (irreversible dilatation of bronchi following damage to the bronchial wall) or cystic fibrosis.

The colour of the sputum may suggest a cause. Infection is often indicated by yellow/green sputum that contains polymorphonuclear leucocytes (pus cells). In allergic conditions such as asthma, sputum is only rarely infected, but is often discoloured yellow/green by eosinophils. White frothy sputum is a feature of pulmonary oedema.

Common causes of bloodstained sputum (haemoptysis)

- Pneumonia;
- bronchial carcinoma;
- pulmonary embolism;
- pulmonary oedema (frothy bloodstained sputum);
- pulmonary tuberculosis (TB);
- pulmonary vasculitis.

Haemoptysis may also be caused by other tumours of the respiratory tract (e.g. of the nasopharynx, larynx) or by trauma.

Dyspnoea (History box 6, p. 9)

Dyspnoea means difficulty in breathing, and is a feature of lower respiratory tract disease.

History box 6
Questions to ask about dyspnoea

When did it start?
How often does it occur? — is it intermittent (asthma, bronchitis)? persistent?
Are there any associated features? — chest pain? pleuritic pain? productive cough? haemoptysis? fever? wheeze?
Does anything bring it on? — allergens? cold? exercise?
Do you work with chemicals, dyes, dust?
Is breathing more difficult when you lie flat (orthopnoea)?
Do you wake gasping for breath at night (paroxysmal nocturnal dyspnoea)?
How many pillows do you use to prop yourself up at night?

1

Common causes of dyspnoea

- Bronchitis and pneumonia;
- asthma;
- pulmonary oedema due to left ventricular failure;
- infiltration of the lungs (usually carcinomatous).

Dyspnoea is intermittent in asthma and bronchitis, but persistent and progressively worse if due to lung infiltrates (carcinomatosis, fibrosing alveolitis). Associated features include fever if caused by an infection, a wheeze in asthma, and haemoptysis and pleuritic pain in pulmonary embolism.

Allergens, cold and exercise can all induce asthma. Occupational asthma may follow exposure to various allergens including wood dusts, cotton, platinum salts (used in refining), and dyes and chemicals used in printing. Symptoms improve at weekends and during holidays. The allergic response of occupational exposure may also cause interstitial pulmonary fibrosis.

Orthopnoea

Orthopnoea is breathlessness on lying flat. In this position the accessory respiratory muscles are impaired and abdominal pressure is increased, impeding movement of the diaphragm. Breathlessness from any cause is therefore aggravated by lying flat.

In heart failure, pooling of blood in the lungs from weakness of the cardiac pump is aggravated by increased venous return of blood (normally pooled in the lower limbs). Orthopnoea and attacks of breathlessness during the night (paroxysmal nocturnal dyspnoea) are therefore particularly common in heart failure.

History box 7
Questions to ask about palpitations

When did the palpitations start?
How long do they last?
Are they persistent or intermittent?
Do they start and stop suddenly?
Are there any associated features? — chest pain? syncope? anxiety? thyrotoxicosis?
Are there any relieving factors?

Palpitations (History box 7, above)

Palpitation implies awareness of the heart beat, which can be variably described as 'palpitations', 'the heart missing a beat', 'rapid heart beat' or 'fluttering in the chest'.

Common causes of palpitations

Ectopic beats (extrasystoles) Common and usually unrelated to underlying heart disease. Can be either atrial ectopics (arising in the atria from a site other than the sinoatrial (SA) node) or ventricular ectopics (arising in the ventricles).

Sinus tachycardia Arises from the sinus node (often related to anxiety or excessive intake of caffeine or nicotine, but may be due to thyrotoxicosis or systemic illness if persistent).

Arrhythmia (see pp. 64 and 303–6) An abnormality of cardiac rhythm arising in either the *atria* (atrial tachycardia, atrial flutter, atrial fibrillation) or the *ventricles* (ventricular tachycardia).

Arrhythmias may be caused by cardiac, respiratory or systemic diseases. Common cardiac diseases which cause arrhythmias are:

- ischaemic heart disease;
- valvular heart disease;
- cardiomyopathy (p. 167);

- pericarditis.

Respiratory causes include:

- pneumonia;
- pulmonary embolus;
- bronchial carcinoma.

Other causes include:

- thyrotoxicosis;
- septicaemia.

Palpitations are rarely described as persistent because patient awareness is usually intermittent, even in the presence of a persisting arrhythmia such as atrial fibrillation.

Palpitations that start and stop suddenly are a feature of paroxysmal atrial or ventricular tachycardia.

Associated features may include chest pain, if the palpitations are due to cardiac ischaemia, or syncope, if associated with low cardiac output. Other features to look for are those of thyrotoxicosis (pp. 206–7), which may cause atrial fibrillation, and anxiety.

Atrial tachycardias may be relieved by increasing vagal tone, using either carotid sinus pressure or the Valsalva manoeuvre (forced expiration against a closed glottis).

Chest pain (History box 2, p. 4)

Chest pain may arise from any of the thoracic viscera (Fig. 1.1, p. 15). The common types are detailed in Information box 1 on pp. 12–14, and include angina (ischaemic cardiac pain), myocardial infarction (heart attack or heart muscle death), oesophageal acid reflux, musculoskeletal strain, pleurisy (irritation of the parietal pleura), and pericarditis (irritation of the pericardium). Cardiac and oesophageal pain can be difficult to distinguish.

Ischaemic heart disease

This is usually caused by atheromatous narrowing of the coronary arteries which predisposes to formation of a thrombus (blood clot rich in platelets and neutrophils), resulting in occlusion of the artery and myocardial infarction. Rarer causes include coronary artery spasm, coronary artery emboli (fragments, usually of thrombi, which travel in the bloodstream from their

Information box 1
Types of chest pain

Angina

Site	Central chest
Onset	May be recent or have been occurring, on and off, for many years
Character	Tight, crushing or band-like
Radiation	To arms and neck
Associations	Patient often gestures using a clenched fist in front of the sternum
Timing	Intermittent, often with clear relation to exacerbating factors
Exacerbating factors	Induced by exercise, particularly if it is cold weather, and sometimes by emotion or a heavy meal
Relieving factors	Relieved by rest and glyceryl trinitrate (GTN)
Severity	Variable

Myocardial infarction

Similar pain to that of angina, but lasts longer and is more severe
Often associated with sweating, nausea and vomiting, and fear

Oesophageal acid reflux

Site	Retrosternal
Onset	Common after meals, and on bending or lying flat
Character	Burning, sore
Radiation	May radiate to back or be associated with epigastric pain or discomfort
Associations	Usually associated with a lot of flatulence, particularly if antacid therapy is used
Timing	Often occurs at night (particularly after a large meal)
Exacerbating factors	Induced by lying flat, bending, lifting and eating certain foods – often fried or spicy foods, but this varies according to the patient

Relieving factors   Relieved by antacids
Severity   Varies from mild discomfort to severe pain (can be indistinguishable from myocardial infarction)

Pleurisy
Site   Usually felt at specific area of inflammation
Onset   Often sudden
Character   Sharp, knife-like
Radiation   Usually localized without radiation
Associations   Breathlessness, cough, sputum or haemoptysis suggest underlying lung problem such as pulmonary embolus
Timing   Continuous with sharp exacerbations
Exacerbating factors Aggravated by inspiration and coughing
Relieving factors
Severity   Variable

Pericarditis
Site   Central chest
Onset   May follow myocardial infarction or viral infection
Character   Sore or pressing
Radiation   Often none. May radiate to neck or shoulders
Associations   Fever is common, irrespective of cause. May be symptoms of viral infection
Timing   During the first few days after myocardial infarction. At the time of, or following, viral infection
Exacerbating factors Aggravated by posture (usually lying flat) and respiration
Relieving factors
Severity   Variable

Continued overleaf

1

Information box 1 *Contd*

Musculoskeletal pain

Site	Any site
Onset	Follows unusual muscular activity
Character	Aching
Radiation	Often none, but depends on site
Associations	Local tenderness
Timing	Often recurs at the same site
Exacerbating factors	Aggravated by movement
Relieving factors	Relieved by rest and local heat
Severity	Variable

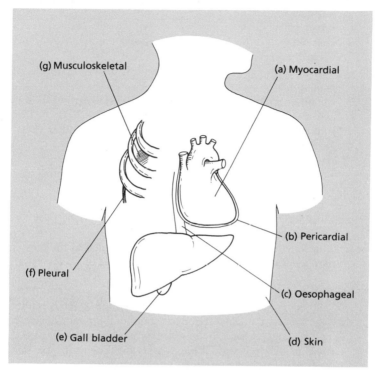

Fig. 1.1 Types of chest pain. (a) Myocardial — tight, crushing central chest pain. Radiates to arms, neck. Induced by exercise, emotion, cold. Relieved by rest, GTN. (b) Pericardial — sore or pressing central chest pain. Changes with posture. (c) Oesophageal — retrosternal, sore or burning. Worse on bending, lying flat. Eased by antacids. (d) Skin — herpes zoster (pain may precede rash). (e) Gall bladder — pain below right costal margin, referred to right shoulder. Very tender to pressure. (f) Pleural — sharp, 'knife-like' pain on inspiration. (g) Musculoskeletal — sore or 'catching' on movement. Usually localized tenderness.

site of origin to lodge in and occlude vessels at distant sites), or reduced delivery of oxygen to the myocardium due to anaemia, carboxyhaemoglobinaemia or hypotension.

Causes of oesophageal acid reflux
- Hiatus hernia;

- obesity;
- pregnancy;
- smoking.

Causes of pleurisy

- Infection (viral or in association with underlying bacterial pneumonia);
- pulmonary embolism (implying infarction of peripheral lung and usually associated with haemoptysis);
- infiltration (spread of cancer from the lung or other sites);
- connective tissue disease.*

Causes of pericarditis

- Infection (usually viral but may be bacterial including TB);
- myocardial infarction or cardiac surgery;
- malignant infiltration;
- connective tissue disease;
- severe uraemia.

Questions to ask about chest pain are outlined in the master plan for pain (SOCRATES) in History box 2 on p. 4.

Ankle oedema (History box 8, p. 17)

Ankle oedema is caused by the collection of fluid in extravascular tissues due to either obstruction of venous or lymphatic drainage, or failure to retain fluid in the vascular compartment because of reduced oncotic pressure. It presents as swelling of the feet and ankles, which may progress to involve the calves and thighs and, in severe cases, the trunk.

Common causes of ankle oedema

- Venous congestion (e.g. due to right heart failure);
- deep venous thrombosis (DVT — clots in the deep leg veins);
- lymphatic obstruction (e.g. due to lymph node infiltration by lymphoma or tumour);
- low oncotic pressure (due to a low serum albumin in chronic liver disease, nephrotic syndrome or malnutrition).

---

* The term 'connective tissue disease' has evolved to describe a group of inflammatory conditions, such as systemic lupus erythematosus (SLE) and rheumatoid arthritis, in which there is multiple organ involvement. The term is widely used, although it is misleading as the target of the inflammatory process is often not connective tissue.

History box 8
Questions to ask about ankle swelling

When did the swelling start?
Do both legs swell?
Is it worse at any particular time during the day?
Have you had any pain in the calves or legs?
Do you suffer from a cough or breathlessness?
Do you have any history of kidney or liver problems?
Have you noticed any change in your urine?

Usually the swelling is worse towards the end of the day and after prolonged standing, which increases the hydrostatic pressure.

Oedema due to venous congestion or low oncotic pressure is 'pitting' oedema (i.e. slow gentle pressure for 5 seconds leaves a pit or hollow in the skin) and usually improves overnight or whilst resting with the legs elevated.

Long-standing oedema due to lymphatic obstruction does not pit or vary with time of day or position.

Gastrointestinal symptoms

The commonest gastrointestinal disorders are:
• infective gastroenteritis;
• oesophageal reflux;
• constipation, especially in the elderly;
• peptic ulceration (ulceration arising in or near pepsin- and acid-secreting mucosa);
• gastric carcinoma;
• irritable bowel syndrome;
• diverticular disease;
• colorectal carcinoma.
Ulcerative colitis and Crohn's disease are common in hospital practice.

Appetite (History box 9, p. 18)
Increased appetite is a feature of thyrotoxicosis.

Loss of appetite (anorexia) occurs with most serious illnesses,

History box 9
Questions to ask about appetite and weight

Have you been eating more or less recently?
Do you have any soreness of the mouth or tongue?
Do you have any difficulty swallowing?
Have you suffered from any nausea or vomiting?
Have you noticed any change in your weight?
Do you have any abdominal pain?

but particularly with disorders of the upper gut (gastritis, peptic ulceration, gastric carcinoma), anxiety and depression.

Soreness of the tongue (glossitis) or mouth (stomatitis) may cause marked anorexia and dysphagia.

Causes of glossitis and stomatitis
- Ill-fitting dentures;
- infections — *bacterial* (e.g. anaerobes, often in association with poor dental hygiene), *viral* (e.g herpes simplex with recurrent herpes labialis or cold sores; Coxsackie A causing oral ulceration with a rash on the hands, feet and buttocks), *fungal* (e.g. *Candida albicans* — thrush);
- recurrent aphthous ulceration — recurrent painful superficial ulcers of unknown cause;
- inflammatory bowel disease (Crohn's, ulcerative colitis, p. 180);
- coeliac disease (p. 181);
- vitamin deficiencies including iron, folate and B_{12}.

Weight (History box 9, above)

Weight gain is usually a result of overeating and, less commonly, hypothyroidism and fluid retention in cardiac, renal or liver failure. Weight gain during corticosteroid therapy may result from appetite stimulation or fluid retention (a mineralocorticoid effect).

Weight loss accompanies most serious illnesses, particularly if associated with anorexia or nausea. It may be the presenting feature of underlying malignancy.

Thyrotoxicosis produces the unique combination of increased appetite and weight loss.

Nausea and vomiting (History box 10, p. 20)

Nausea and vomiting are caused by gastrointestinal (oesophageal, gastric, duodenal, small bowel), neurological (usually vestibular) or metabolic disease.

Causes of nausea and vomiting (Common causes are in *italics*)

Oesophageal causes
- *Oesophageal acid reflux with oesophagitis;*
- *oesophageal ulceration;*
- hiatus hernia (herniation of the stomach through the diaphragm);
- oesophageal carcinoma.

Gastric causes
- *Gastritis due to infectious food poisoning* (the most common cause);
- *alcohol-induced gastritis;*
- *drug-induced gastritis* (many drugs, including alcohol, aspirin, non-steroidal anti-inflammatory drugs and corticosteroids);
- *gastric ulceration;*
- gastric carcinoma;
- pyloric stenosis (in adults usually due to scarring and oedema from ulceration, in children due to congenital hyperplasia of the pylorus).

Duodenal and small bowel causes
- *Duodenitis;*
- *duodenal ulceration;*
- small bowel obstruction.

Neurological causes
- *Motion sickness;*
- acute labyrinthitis;
- Menierè's disease (p. 34).

Metabolic causes
- Diabetic ketoacidosis;
- uraemia (nausea may be the presenting feature of chronic renal failure);
- hypercalcaemia.

History box 10
Questions to ask about nausea, vomiting and haematemesis

Questions to ask about nausea and vomiting
When did the symptoms start?
Do you have any other abdominal symptoms?
What medicines do you take?
Do you drink alcohol? – if so what? how much? how often?
Do you smoke? (prevents healing of peptic ulcers)
Do you ever feel as though the room is spinning (vertigo) or suffer from deafness?
Do you have any history of kidney problems?

Questions to ask about haematemesis
What was the appearance of the vomited blood?
How much did you vomit – a spoonful? a cupful? half a pint?
Do you have any chest or abdominal pain or discomfort?
What medicines do you take? – have you been taking aspirin? other pain killers? corticosteroids?
How much alcohol do you drink?

Other causes
- *Pregnancy*;
- *drugs*, including most used in cancer chemotherapy;
- infections, particularly urinary infections in children and the elderly.

Haematemesis (History box 10, p. 20)

Haematemesis is vomiting of blood. The vomited blood may be fresh or clotted, or may have been digested by gastric acid to produce a brown fluid like coffee grounds. (Blood from the lungs is bright red and often mixed with sputum.)

Causes of haematemesis (In order of frequency)
- Gastric erosion;
- oesophagitis and Mallory−Weiss tears (i.e tears of the oesophageal mucosa after forceful vomiting);
- duodenal ulcer;
- gastric ulcer;
- oesophageal varices (dilated oesophageal veins due to portal venous hypertension).

Vomiting of fresh blood implies recent bleeding. The presence of blood is alarming to the patient and the quantity may be overestimated. It is important to ask about alcohol consumption because it is associated with peptic ulceration and liver disease with portal varices.

Dysphagia (History box 11, p. 22)

Dysphagia means difficulty in swallowing, and may be considered anatomically in terms of disease of the mouth and tongue, oropharynx, oesophagus and upper stomach.

The patient will be aware of food sticking. The site of obstruction is often thought to be higher than the lesion, and is impossible to determine from the history alone.

Any marked weight loss suggests an underlying carcinoma of oesophagus or stomach, whereas recurrent chest infections are common in achalasia due to overspill from the oesophagus into the lungs.

Although dysphagia is a common psychological symptom — usually of anxiety — it must always be taken seriously and investigated, and never disregarded.

History box 11
Questions to ask about dysphagia

Do you have more difficulty swallowing liquids or solids?
Where does food stick?
Do you vomit food back, and if so is it easily recognizable (i.e. has it reached the stomach and been digested)?
Is there any associated pain?
Have you suffered previously from chest or abdominal pain or discomfort?
Have you noticed any weight loss?
Do you have any chest problems?

Patients with obstructive lesions (e.g. oesophageal carcinoma) experience more difficulty swallowing solids (which stick at the obstruction) compared with liquids. Patients with neurological problems affecting the palate (e.g. strokes or bulbar palsy — p. 127) often have more difficulty swallowing liquids, which easily regurgitate into the trachea.

Causes of dysphagia

Common causes are:
- tonsillitis and pharyngitis (the most common cause);
- benign oesophageal stricture (usually due to reflux oesophagitis);
- stroke;
- oesophageal carcinoma;
- gastric carcinoma.

Rarer causes are:
- achalasia of the cardia (a neuromuscular disorder affecting the motility of the entire oesophagus);
- pharyngeal pouch;
- external pressure on the oesophagus due to bronchial carcinoma, retrosternal goitre, enlarged left atrium or thoracic aortic aneurysm;
- Plummer–Vinson (Paterson–Kelly) syndrome (the association of iron-deficiency anaemia and a pre-cancerous post-cricoid web);
- neurological disease (e.g. myasthenia gravis, bulbar palsy), when dysphagia is often greater for liquids than for solids;
- scleroderma.

Acute abdominal pain

It is important to distinguish between the recent pain (hours or days) of an 'acute abdomen' and longer-standing pain (weeks or months) of a 'chronic abdomen'.

As with all pain ask questions about abdominal pain according to the master plan (SOCRATES) shown in History box 2 on p. 4.

The acute (surgical) abdomen is characterized by severe abdominal pain of short duration, usually in a previously well individual. The common causes of abdominal pain are listed below. The usual sites of these pains and their characteristic features are shown in Fig. 1.2.

Common causes of acute abdominal pain
- Intestinal infection (usually food poisoning);
- appendicitis;
- duodenal or gastric ulceration, with or without perforation;
- diverticulitis (inflammation in an outpouching of the bowel wall — a diverticulum);
- intestinal obstruction;
- biliary colic (impaction of gallstones in the neck of the gall bladder or cystic duct);
- cholecystitis (inflammation in the gall bladder, usually in association with gallstones);
- pancreatitis;
- urinary infection;
- ureteric colic (impaction of a kidney stone in the ureter);
- gynaecological disorders — dysmenorrhea, ovarian cyst, ectopic pregnancy.

Peritonitis

Peritonitis means inflammation of the peritoneum. It occurs locally with any inflammatory condition (e.g. appendicitis, diverticulitis, cholecystitis). Following rupture of a hollow intra-abdominal viscus (e.g. perforation of the appendix, a duodenal ulcer or a colonic diverticulum), it becomes more severe and generalized, and is associated with spread of infection through the peritoneum.

Less commonly, peritonitis is due to a chemical (enzymatic) inflammation as a result of acute pancreatitis releasing enzymes into the peritoneal cavity.

The main clinical features of peritonitis are severe generalized abdominal pain in a patient who lies still to prevent it. There is tenderness on minimal abdominal pressure, and rebound tenderness — pain on lifting the examining hand quickly from the abdomen.

Chronic abdominal pain

Chronic abdominal pain is usually intermittent and of longer duration than that of an acute abdomen.

Common causes of chronic abdominal pain

Peptic ulceration Ulceration occurring in proximity to acid-

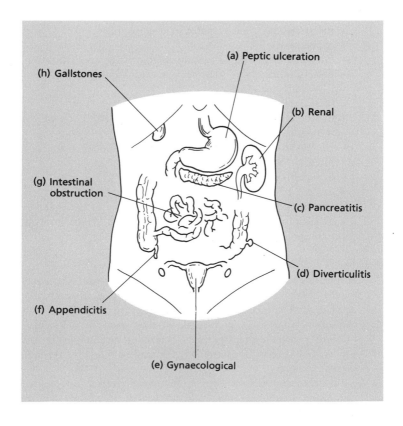

(a) Peptic ulceration

(h) Gallstones

(b) Renal

(g) Intestinal obstruction

(c) Pancreatitis

(d) Diverticulitis

(f) Appendicitis

(e) Gynaecological

producing areas of the gastrointestinal tract; most commonly stomach or proximal duodenum, but also at other sites including oesophagus or a Meckel's diverticulum, an out-pouching of the ileum containing ectopic gastric mucosa, which is found in 2% of the population.

May present as an acute abdomen.

Usually gives rise to epigastric pain occurring in attacks lasting days or weeks, interspersed with periods of relief.

Pain is often related to meals, relieved by antacids, and may be associated with nausea and vomiting.

May bleed, causing haematemesis and/or melaena and perforate causing peritonitis.

Irritable bowel syndrome Spasm or abnormal motility of the bowel in the absence of organic pathology may cause abdominal pain at any site.

Often associated with abdominal distension ('bloatedness') and changes in bowel habit.

Fig. 1.2 (*Opposite.*) Usual sites of different abdominal pains. (a) Peptic ulceration — intermittent epigastric pain, often related to meals, eased by antacids. *Perforation* — severe generalized pain aggravated by movement. (b) Renal. *Pyelonephritis* (infection within kidney) — loin pain, dysuria and urinary frequency. *Ureteric colic* (impaction of stone in urinary tract) — severe pain with sharp exacerbations, radiating to groin. (c) Pancreatitis — severe, constant epigastric pain radiating to back with vomiting. (d) Diverticulitis (infection in colonic diverticulum) — commonest in descending colon. Central pain moving to left iliac fossa, usually with altered bowel habit and sometimes rectal bleeding. (e) Gynaecological — lower abdominal pain with or without menstrual disturbance or vaginal discharge in women. Consider pelvic inflammatory disease, twisted/ruptured ovarian cyst, ectopic pregnancy, endometriosis. (f) Appendicitis — central abdominal pain shifting to the right iliac fossa. Aggravated by movement, associated with anorexia, nausea and vomiting. (g) Intestinal obstruction — colicky pain with vomiting, abdominal distension and absolute constipation (faeces and flatus) if complete obstruction. (h) Gallstones — impaction in the gall bladder neck or biliary ducts (biliary colic) with or without inflammation (cholecystitis). Right upper quadrant pain radiating to right shoulder, usually accompanied by vomiting.

Gallstones Repeated episodes of inflammation in the gall bladder (cholecystitis), associated in over 90% of cases with the presence of gallstones.

Causes right subcostal pain referred to the right shoulder.

Discomfort may occur after fatty meals, which stimulate gall bladder contraction, and be associated with nausea and flatulence.

Gallstones are commoner in women and associated with obesity, use of oral contraceptives and increasing age. However, they occur in 10–20% of the general population – the concept that they only occur in fair, fat, fertile, females of forty is misleading.

Diverticular disease A diverticulum is an outpouching of mucosa between hypertrophied muscle, usually in the sigmoid colon.

May cause painful diverticular disease – probably due to abnormal bowel motility – or diverticulitis (inflammation around a diverticulum).

Pain is usually in the left iliac fossa, or across the lower abdomen, and is associated with alteration in bowel habit.

Inflammatory bowel disease Abdominal pain in Crohn's disease and ulcerative colitis is associated with altered bowel habit, rectal bleeding and generalized systemic symptoms of malaise, fever, anorexia and weight loss.

Gynaecological disease Lower abdominal pain in women with or without menstrual disturbance or vaginal discharge.

May be caused by pelvic infection, an ovarian cyst or endometriosis. Ectopic pregnancy can be excluded by a negative pregnancy test or confirmed by ultrasound.

Questions to ask As with all pain, ask questions about chronic abdominal pain according to the master plan (SOCRATES) shown in History box 2 on p. 4.

Bowel action and frequency (History box 12, p. 27)

Most people fall into the range three in 1 day to 1 in 3 days, but there is no normal bowel action as the range of normality varies from three to four times daily to once per week. When enquiring about bowel habit, it is a change from normal which is significant.

History box 12
Questions to ask about bowel action and frequency, and rectal bleeding

Questions to ask about bowel action and frequency
Has there been any change in your bowel action or its frequency?
Do you pass any mucus or blood with your bowel action?

Questions to ask about rectal bleeding
When did the bleeding start?
Is the blood on the surface of the stool or on the paper or mixed with the stool?
Have you had any pain on defaecation?
Have you had any abdominal pain?
Is there any mucus?
Have you been travelling abroad?

Causes of increased frequency of loose bowel actions (diarrhoea)
- Infective gastroenteritis;
- anxiety;
- irritable bowel syndrome;
- diverticulitis;
- drugs (antibiotics alter bowel flora, purgatives).

Less commonly diarrhoea is due to malabsorption, inflammatory bowel disease (ulcerative colitis and Crohn's disease), thyrotoxicosis, or opportunistic infection (e.g. *Cryptosporidium*) of the gut in human immunodeficiency virus (HIV) infection.

Causes of decreased frequency of bowel actions (constipation)
There is usually no obvious underlying cause of constipation, but it may be associated with:
- depression;
- painful anal lesions (piles and fissures);
- drugs (analgesics);
- dehydration;
- hypothyroidism.

Absolute constipation for flatus and faeces implies bowel obstruction. Intermittent change of bowel habit, particularly in the over-50s, suggests intermittent obstruction by carcinoma of the colon.

Stools

Causes of abnormal stools Melaena, the passage of black 'tarry' stools with a characteristic smell, results from the digestion of blood, usually by gastric acid, and indicates bleeding from the upper gastrointestinal tract — invariably above the ileocaecal valve. Iron tablets also make stools black and tarry.

Putty-coloured stools are produced in the absence of bile pigment, as occurs in obstructive jaundice. Pale, offensive and bulky stools that do not flush easily are a feature of malabsorption.

Rectal bleeding

Causes of rectal bleeding The most common cause of rectal bleeding is haemorrhoids (piles). Other common causes are:
- rectal or colonic polyps or carcinoma;
- diverticular disease;
- infective colitis;
- inflammatory bowel disease (ulcerative colitis and Crohn's disease);
- anal fissure.

Questions to ask about rectal bleeding are listed in History box 12 on p. 27, and the answers can give helpful diagnostic clues:
- bright red blood on the surface of the stool or on the paper suggests piles or anal fissure;
- pain on defaecation is a feature of anal fissure;
- alteration in bowel habit is characteristic of colorectal carcinoma;
- abdominal pain is a feature of dysentery, inflammatory bowel disease or diverticular disease;
- the presence of mucus suggests inflammatory bowel disease or carcinoma;
- foreign travel suggests amoebic colitis or dysentery.

Genitourinary symptoms

Dysuria (History box 13, p. 29)

Dysuria is pain or burning on micturition felt in the urethra,

1

History box 13
Questions to ask about dysuria and haematuria

Questions to ask about dysuria
Have you had pain passing urine before?
Have you passed any blood, gravel or stones?
Do you have any penile/vaginal discharge?
What sexual contacts have you had? — when? with what contraception?
   with whom (contact tracing)?
Was (were) your partner(s) male or female?

Questions to ask about haematuria
As for dysuria *plus*:
Is blood present throughout or at the end of micturition?
Do you have any loin or abdominal pain?
Do you have a family history of kidney disease?

---

often with suprapubic pain. It implies inflammation of the urethral or bladder mucosa.

Common causes of dysuria

- Urinary tract infection;
- urethritis (gonococcal, non-specific);
- prostatitis;
- urinary tract stones.

Difficulty starting micturition, poor stream and dribbling at the end of micturition in men are symptoms of prostatic hypertrophy.

Haematuria (History box 13, above)

The passage of blood on micturition.

Causes of haematuria

- Urinary tract infection;
- urinary tract stones;
- urothelial tumours;
- renal tumours.

Less common causes are polycystic kidneys and glomerulonephritis, trauma to the kidneys or urinary tract, and coagulation disorders.

The presence of blood throughout micturition suggests a lesion of the upper urinary tract (kidneys), whereas the passage of blood at the end of micturition suggests a lower urinary tract lesion (bladder).

Loin pain

Loin pain can be a feature of a renal stone or a renal tumour; ureteric colic (severe intermittent loin or abdominal pain due to intermittent ureteric obstruction) can be caused by stones or a blood clot which obstructs the flow of urine.

Penile discharge (History box 13, p. 29)

A urethral discharge usually indicates a sexually transmitted infection.

Common causes of penile discharge

- Gonorrhoea;
- non-specific urethritis (non-gonococcal infection, often due to *Trichomonas vaginalis*, *Candida albicans*, *Mycoplasma*, *Chlamydia*).

Gynaecological symptoms (History box 14, p. 31)

Amenorrhoea

An absence of periods (amenorrhoea) may be primary (i.e. never begun) because the patient is too young or because of anovulation (due to hypothalamic–pituitary disorders) or ovarian agenesis (as in Turner's syndrome).

Secondary amenorrhoea

Secondary amenorrhoea (i.e. cessation of periods after a normal menarche) results from pregnancy, anorexia nervosa or any debilitating illness. Rarely it is due to either a pituitary lesion (e.g. tumour or infarction) or polycystic ovaries.

Menorrhagia

Heavy or prolonged menstrual bleeding (menorrhagia) is usually associated with uterine fibroids.

Uterine or cervical carcinoma

Uterine or cervical carcinoma is suggested by post-menopausal vaginal bleeding.

History box 14
Questions to ask about gynaecological symptoms

Questions to ask about amenorrhoea
Have you ever had any menstrual bleeding?
If so, at what age did your periods start?
Were they regular, and when did they stop?
Have you had any pregnancies?
Have you taken the contraceptive pill?

Questions to ask about menorrhagia
How often do your periods occur?
How many days do they last?
Do you pass clots?
Are your periods heavy?

Questions to ask about post-menopausal vaginal bleeding
When did the bleeding start?
When did your periods finish?
How often and how heavy is the bleeding?
Have you had any vaginal discharge?
Have you had any abdominal or pelvic pain?

Questions to ask about vaginal discharge
What colour is the discharge?
Have you had any vaginal irritation?
Do you have any pain on intercourse (dyspareunia)?
Have you had any recent sexual contact?

Vaginal discharge

A vaginal discharge of fluid (serous or pus) usually indicates infection with *Candida albicans*, which is usually associated with intense vaginal irritation, *Trichomonas vaginalis* or, more rarely, gonococcus.

Dyspareunia

Dyspareunia (pain on intercourse) occurs with inflammation or infection of the vulva, urethra, vagina or cervix, following episiotomy, and with pelvic lesions such as endometriosis or malignancy (e.g. ovarian or uterine). Vaginal atrophy is a common cause in post-menopausal women. Psychological causes should also be considered.

Neurological symptoms

Headache (History box 2, p. 4)

Headache is the commonest neurological symptom — and perhaps the most common symptom of all.

Causes of headache

Tension headache The commonest type of headache; usually bilateral and often involving occipital, temporal or frontal musculature.

Often an obvious association with stress.

Vomiting is not a feature.

The description is often dramatic — 'like a screwdriver going in here'.

Sinusitis Sinus infection may cause localized pain in the face, in the upper jaw or behind the eyes.

Toothache Infected or impacted teeth may cause pain in the jaw or face.

Migraine Typically there is a prodromal aura (feeling which precedes and heralds the onset of an attack) with visual disturbance (e.g. partial loss of vision or flashing lights) due to arterial spasm causing intracranial ischaemia. This is followed by severe unilateral headache, vomiting, and photophobia (marked discomfort looking at light) due to intracranial arterial vasodilatation. Occasionally unilateral signs, which recover within 24 hours, develop.

Rare important causes are:
- cranial arteritis;
   inflammation of any of the cranial arteries, but often of the temporal arteries;
   usually affects the elderly;
   causes pain and local tenderness;
   ophthalmic artery involvement may cause visual loss;
- cerebral tumour;
   the headache of raised intracranial pressure is worse in the morning and associated with vomiting and often visual blurring (see papilloedema, pp. 114 and 116);
- meningeal irritation;
   gives rise to severe generalized headache with neck stiffness, vomiting and photophobia;

due either to extravasated blood (subarachnoid haemorrhage), when the onset is usually sudden, or to infection (meningitis);

- trigeminal neuralgia;
  causes severe shooting facial pain in the distribution of the trigeminal nerve with 'trigger points' — 'it occurs when I touch or brush my cheek'.

History box 15
Questions to ask about blackouts, dizziness and vertigo

Questions to ask about blackouts
When did you have your first blackout? — have you had them throughout your life? or are they of recent onset?
How often do they occur?
What have you been doing when they occur?
For how long are you unconscious?
Do you have any warning that they are going to occur (prodromal aura)?
Do you jerk your limbs, bite your tongue or become incontinent?
Do you have any palpitations or chest pain?
Do you notice any hunger and sweating?
Are the blackouts associated with coughing or passing urine?

Questions to ask about dizziness and vertigo
When did the dizziness start?
Does anything bring it on?
Do you feel your head spinning during attacks (vertigo)?
Do you suffer from nausea or vomiting during attacks?
Do you have any hearing problems?

Blackouts (History box 15, above)

Blackouts may be caused by cardiovascular, cerebral or metabolic disease.

Cardiovascular causes (resulting in reduced cerebral blood flow)

- Faint (vasovagal attack);
- arrhythmias — either tachycardias (atrial or ventricular) or bradycardias (e.g. complete heart block);
- aortic stenosis;

- postural hypotension (e.g. due to dehydration, or loss of the normal sympathetic nervous responses to standing in autonomic nerve dysfunction);
- drugs (e.g. diuretics, antihypertensives).

Cerebral causes
- Epilepsy (see pp. 193–4);
- transient ischaemic attack (TIA);
- stroke (cerebral infarction or haemorrhage);
- trauma (head injury).

Metabolic cause
- Hypoglycaemia (due to too much insulin, insufficient carbohydrate or excessive exercise in diabetics, or very rarely insulinoma).

NB: A prodromal aura (strange sensation, noise or discomfort), jerking limbs, tongue biting or incontinence suggests an epileptic attack.

Hunger and sweating suggest hypoglycaemia, which may be accompanied by confusion and aggression if severe.

Increased vagal tone and interference with the venous return to the heart whilst straining during coughing or micturition may cause fainting in the elderly (cough or micturition syncope).

Anyone who has had a blackout should lie in the coma position for about 4–10 minutes until recovered, otherwise the period of unconsciousness may be prolonged and can end with a fit.

Dizziness and vertigo (History box 15, p. 33)

Causes Dizziness is common, particularly in the elderly. It refers to the sensation of instability and rarely indicates serious underlying disease. True vertigo (a sensation of rotation) indicates a disturbance of the inner ear or its connections (i.e. eighth cranial nerve, brain stem or cerebellum).

The commonest cause of vertigo is acute labyrinthitis. Rare causes are: posterior fossa tumours, acoustic neuroma, cerebellar tumours, brain stem lesions, drugs and Menière's disease.

In Menière's disease increased fluid pressure in the inner ear causes attacks of deafness, tinnitus, vertigo and vomiting.

History box 16
Questions to ask about hearing, smell and vision

Questions to ask about hearing
Do you have any difficulty hearing?
Are one or both ears affected?
Have you ever suffered a head injury?
Do you have any ringing in the ears?
Do you suffer from dizziness?

Questions to ask about smell
Have you noticed any change in your sense of smell?

Questions to ask about vision
Do you have any problems with your vision?
Does it affect one eye or both?
When did you first notice the problem?
Do you wear glasses?
Have you had any pain or irritation in the eye?

Hearing (History box 16, above)
Common causes of hearing loss
- Ear wax;
- progressive loss of eighth nerve function with increasing age (presbycusis);
- middle ear infection (otitis media).

Rarer causes are: trauma involving the inner ear or eighth nerve, brain stem lesions, drugs (quinine, aspirin, aminoglycosides) or acoustic neuroma.

An altered or heightened auditory acuity (hyperacusis) may be a feature of temporal lobe epilepsy (rare) or of a seventh nerve lesion involving the nerve to stapedius (very rare).

Tinnitus
Tinnitus is ringing in the ear, and indicates a lesion of the inner ear which may be associated with deafness and vertigo.

Common causes include: infection, drugs (e.g. aspirin) and Menière's disease.

Smell (History box 16, p. 35)

Common causes of loss of smell
- Sinusitis;
- upper respiratory infection.

Rarer causes include compression of the olfactory nerve by tumour (e.g. olfactory groove meningioma) or trauma associated with fracture of the cribriform plate.

An altered or heightened sensation of smell is rare, but may occur with temporal lobe epilepsy.

Taste

Causes of abnormal taste The common causes of a diminished sensation of taste are:
- sinusitis;
- upper respiratory infection.

Rarer causes include brain stem lesions affecting the fifth or ninth cranial nerve nuclei.

Strange tastes are caused by drugs, which may be excreted in the saliva (e.g. metronidazole), renal failure, hepatic failure or temporal lobe epilepsy (rare). The symptom is not uncommon, and often no cause is found.

Vision (History box 16, p. 35)

Common causes of diminished vision or blindness
- Refractive errors — short sight (myopia), long sight (hypermetropia);
- cataracts;
- glaucoma;
- diabetic retinopathy.

Poorly controlled diabetes mellitus may cause varying changes in the intraocular glucose concentration, resulting in temporary refractive errors.

Rarer causes of diminution or loss of vision include: optic neuritis, vitreous haemorrhage, detached retina (sudden loss of vision) or occipital lesions (very rare). A patient with cortical blindness (due to bilateral occipital lobe damage involving the optic cortex) may be unaware of their complete loss of vision.

Pituitary tumours may compress the optic chiasma, causing bitemporal hemianopia (loss of both temporal fields of vision with preservation of nasal fields, p. 111).

> **History box 17**
> **Questions to ask about sphincter control and impotence**
>
> **Questions to ask about sphincter control**
> Have you suffered from any incontinence of urine?
> Do you have any other urinary symptoms?
> Is the problem aggravated by coughing or sneezing (stress incontinence)?
> Have you suffered from any incontinence of faeces?
> Has there been any other change in your bowel habit?
>
> **Questions to ask about impotence**
> Do you have difficulty achieving erection, ejaculation or both?
> Do you have early morning erections?

Sphincter control (History box 17, above)

Loss of sphincter control (either bowel or bladder) is rarely a presenting neurological symptom.

Commonest causes of urinary incontinence
- Vaginal prolapse in women;
- prostatic hypertrophy in men.

Faecal incontinence is common in the elderly, due to loss of anal sphincter tone. Constipation, with overflow of loose stools around the impacted faeces, can be an important contributory factor. Other causes include diarrhoea from any cause, rectal prolapse and rectal carcinoma.

Loss of sphincter control also results from lesions of the spinal cord or cauda equina (e.g. spina bifida, compression by external lesions, such as tumours, or demyelination in multiple sclerosis).

Impotence (History box 17, above)

The causes of inability to achieve an erection and ejaculation are often psychological.

Organic causes
- Diabetic autonomic neuropathy;
- drugs (including alcohol);
- spinal cord or cauda equina lesions;
- vascular disease (reduced penile blood flow due to atherosclerosis);

• endocrine disease (hypogonadism as a result of primary gonadal failure, reduced gonadotrophins or hyperprolactinaemia);

• interference with autonomic nerves to the penis during pelvic surgery (abdominoperitoneal resection of the rectum for carcinoma or ulcerative colitis).

History box 18
Questions to ask about muscle weakness

When did the weakness start?
What parts of your body are affected?

Musculoskeletal function

Muscle weakness (History box 18, above)

Causes of muscle weakness may be neurological or myopathic.

Neurological causes The commonest neurological cause is a stroke (cerebrovascular accident (CVA)). A right cerebral haemorrhage or infarct gives rise to weakness in the left lower facial muscles, left arm and left leg. There may be an accompanying sensory loss.

Peripheral nerve lesions cause weakness in the distribution of the muscles supplied and accompanying sensory loss. Causes of peripheral nerve lesions include mononeuropathies and polyneuropathies.

Mononeuropathies These are either isolated or multiple (mononeuritis multiplex, in which there is asymmetrical involvement of several nerves), and include:

• trauma;

• compression (e.g. compression of the median nerve at the wrist in carpal tunnel syndrome — often associated with pregnancy, hypothyroidism, chronic renal failure, rheumatoid arthritis or acromegaly);

• diabetes mellitus;

• connective tissue disease;

- malignancy;
- sarcoidosis;
- leprosy.

Polyneuropathies In polyneuropathies there is usually symmetrical, peripheral neuropathy, often associated with a sensory neuropathy.

Causes of polyneuropathic muscle weakness are:

- metabolic (e.g. diabetes mellitus, uraemia, thyroid disease);
- drugs (e.g. alcohol, vincristine);
- vitamin deficiencies:

    B_1 (beriberi in which polyneuropathy may be associated with cardiomyopathy, and Wernicke's encephalopathy in which ischaemic brain stem damage causes ocular signs, ataxia and confusion);

    B_{12} (peripheral neuropathy may be accompanied by subacute combined degeneration of the cord, in which there is 'combined' demyelination of both lateral (pyramidal) columns, carrying motor fibres, and dorsal (posterior) columns, carrying position and vibration sense and light touch);

- post-infective neuropathy (Guillain–Barré syndrome – motor sensory and sometimes autonomic neuropathy 1–3 weeks after infectious illness; spontaneous recovery invariable, but may take months and be incomplete);

- hereditary neuropathies, such as peroneal muscular atrophy (Charcot–Marie–Tooth disease), in which a slowly progressive, predominantly motor, peripheral neuropathy causes distal muscle weakness and wasting, giving rise in advanced cases to an inverted champagne bottle appearance in the legs.

Myopathic causes of muscle weakness Myopathic weakness due to primary muscle disorders is less common. The causes include:

- muscular dystrophy;
- corticosteroid treatment and Cushing's syndrome, resulting in mainly proximal muscle weakness;
- thyroid disease – mainly proximal muscle weakness;
- osteomalacia – mainly proximal muscle weakness;
- polymyositis – painful proximal muscle weakness due to an inflammatory muscle disorder.

History box 19
Questions to ask about joint pain

Which joints are affected?
How long has the pain been present?
Is it worse on waking?
Does the pain interfere with your activities?

Joint pain (History box 19, above)

Causes The commonest cause of joint pain is osteoarthritis. The incidence increases with age. Any joint may be affected, but large weight-bearing joints, such as knees, hips and the spine, are more commonly involved.

Less commonly, joint pain is due to:

• rheumatoid arthritis, which may affect any joint, although symmetrical involvement of the small joints of the hands is the commonest presentation;

• gout, which is characterized by recurrent exquisite joint pain, usually in the metatarsophalangeal joint of the big toe.

A diagnosis of a septic (infected) arthritis or gout should be considered for any acutely inflamed joint.

Aching pain affecting several joints simultaneously is common in acute infections, such as influenza, rubella (German measles), infectious mononucleosis (glandular fever), *Mycoplasma* pneumonia. It is more rarely a feature of connective tissue disorders (e.g. SLE).

Fleeting and excruciatingly painful arthritis of the joints in children and in teenagers less than 15 years of age occurs in acute rheumatic fever, which is now very rare in the developed world.

Pain in a joint may be referred from other sites — e.g. osteoarthritis in the hip may present with pain in the knee, or cholecystitis may present with pain in the shoulder due to irritation of the diaphragm (innervated by nerve roots C 3, 4, 5, which also supply dermatomes overlying the shoulder).

History box 20
Questions to ask about past medical history

Have you suffered from any previous illness?

Medical
Childhood illness and immunization
Have you had TB or whooping cough?
Have you ever been found to have high blood pressure?
Have you had rheumatic fever?
Have you ever suffered from epileptic seizures?
Do you get asthma (episodic breathlessness, usually with wheeze)?
Have you suffered from anxiety or depression?
Do you have diabetes?

Surgical
Have you had any operations in the past?

Obstetric
Have you had any pregnancies? — were they normal? Were there any
   complications such as hypertension and toxaemia, diabetes, Caesarean
   section?

Aide-mémoire to past medical history (THREAD)
Tuberculosis
Hypertension (myocardial infarction and strokes)
Rheumatic fever
Epilepsy
Asthma, anxiety and arthritis
Diabetes and depression

Past medical history (History box 20, above)

The past medical history gives an overall impression of how fit
the patient has been and may give clues as to the nature of the
current illness.

First ask if the patient has suffered from any previous illness
or undergone any operations. It is then necessary to ask about
specific previous illnesses which may contribute to the current
illness:

• hypertension predisposes to stroke and myocardial
infarction;

- rheumatic fever (now rare in the West) in childhood can lead to adult rheumatic valve disease;
- whooping cough in childhood can cause bronchiectasis and recurrent chest infection;
- TB may become reactivated years after primary infection, particularly in patients who are immunosuppressed;
- long-standing diabetes is associated with vascular disease (stroke, myocardial infarction, peripheral vascular disease), nephropathy, neuropathy and retinopathy;
- gastrectomy for ulcers (now rarely performed since the introduction of H_2-receptor antagonists) can lead to malabsorption;
- psychiatric illness, such as depression or anxiety, can recur and can influence the patient's interpretation of their current illness;
- women should be asked about pregnancies and any complications.

History box 21
Questions to ask about family history

Are your father, mother, brothers, sisters alive? — if they have died, at what age did he/she/they die? What did he/she/they die of?
Do they have any current illnesses?
Do any illnesses run in your family?

Family history (History box 21, above)

Knowledge of illness in the family will help in the overall assessment of the patient's symptoms, which are often partly influenced by worry about a relative or, sometimes, a fear of having the same disease.

Diseases that run in families include:
- hyperlipidaemia (e.g. familial hypercholesterolaemia, familial hypertryglyceridaemia or familial combined hyperlipidaemia);
- angina and myocardial infarction;
- hypertension;
- gastric carcinoma;
- vitamin B_{12} deficiency;

- polycystic kidneys;
- haemoglobinopathies (sickle cell disease, thalassaemia).

Social, occupational and travel history

Questions to ask about social, occupational and travel history are listed in History box 22 (below)

History box 22
Questions to ask about social, occupational and travel history

Who is at home with you?
Are you single, married, widowed or divorced?
Is your partner healthy?
How many children have you got?
Are your children healthy?
What is your occupation?
Do you have any financial worries?
Do you smoke? — if so, how many per day/week?
Have you ever smoked? — why did you give up?
Do you drink alcohol? — if so, how much in units per day/week?
Have you been abroad? — if so, where?
Do you have any pets?
And if mobility is a problem: What is your home like? Do you have to manage stairs? What facilities have you got?

Knowledge of the patient's home situation and facilities is important if the patient has an arthritic, neuromuscular or other disabling disorder. Poor financial circumstances and loneliness make any illness harder to cope with and may be the cause of the presenting problem, but it is often difficult to introduce the topic until you know the patient well.

Travel abroad, especially to tropical and Third World countries, may be accompanied by hepatitis, malaria, dysentery or typhoid.

Well-recognized occupational diseases include:
- asthma (in sensitized workers exposed to wood dusts, cotton, dyes and chemicals);
- pneumoconiosis (due to inhalation of coal dust in miners);
- leptospirosis (infection in vets, farmers and sewer workers

with the spirochaete *Leptospira*, which is excreted in the urine
of rodents);
• anxiety (in anyone who has an insecure job).

Ask about pets and contact with animals (important source of
allergy or infections, such as psittacosis from parrots, *Toxocara*
from dogs and cats).

Drug and therapy history

Questions to ask about drug intake are listed in History box 23
(below).

History box 23
Questions to ask about drug and therapy history

What drugs, homoeopathic and herbal medicines and/or health foods
do you take? — and in what dose?
What other therapies do you have? — physiotherapy? occupational
therapy? malaria prophylaxis?
Do you have any allergies?
Have any medicines ever upset you?

Remember that all drugs have side effects, and many symptoms
are due to drugs. This is particularly true in elderly patients,
who are often taking multiple drugs, which, because of reduced
hepatic metabolism and decreased glomerular filtration, they
excrete more slowly. The risks of dose-dependent side effects
and adverse drug interactions are therefore greatly increased in
the elderly.

Psychiatric assessment (History box 24, pp. 45–6)

About one-third of all patients presenting to their family doctor
have psychiatric problems. Many have obvious psychiatric
symptoms of anxiety or depression and insight into their
symptoms.

Anxiety may be expressed as 'I feel so worried about my
marriage, children, finances'. The person who is depressed may

History box 24
Questions to ask to make a psychiatric assessment

Current symptoms
What are the things that are worrying you?
For each symptom enquire:
When did it start?
How severe is it?
Does it vary?
Ask about the temporal relationship of symptoms to possible
  precipitants such as isolation, interpersonal relationships, work
  environment:
Is it worse or better when you are with other people?
Is it worse or better in certain situations?

Current personal history
Ask about:
Marriage and partners (relationships, social and sexual, and degree of
  satisfaction or concern)
Home situation — who is at home with you?
Relationship with parents and children
Work and money

Current ambitions
Recent disappointments, worries or bereavements of friends and family
Self-esteem
Thought content and abnormal perceptions (suicidal ideas, phobias —
  agoraphobia and claustrophobia, obsession.and compulsive
  behaviour, hallucinations, delusions, depersonalization)

Past family history
Ask about:
Parents and siblings — are relationships in the household happy?
Any history of divorce
Relationship to parents through childhood and adolescence
Relationship to brothers and sisters through childhood and adolescence
Deaths within close family — how was the patient affected?
History of mental disorders and psychiatric diseases

Past personal history
Ask about:
Development and feelings during childhood and adolescence:
• to parents and home

Continued overleaf

History box 24 *Contd*

- to brothers and sisters
- school and teachers with academic and other attainments
- to other people (men, women and friends)

Work satisfaction and achievement including changes and reasons, and ambitions

Previous psychiatric illness, therapy and admissions including alcohol and drug abuse and dependence (e.g. Valium, analgesics, morphine) and convictions if applicable (do not ask about convictions if not appropriate)

Serious illness and particularly head injuries

Points to note while taking the history and while the patient is talking

General appearance including personal response, motor activity, dress, state of agitation

Mood: normal, agitated or depressed

Mental alertness: flow and spontaneity of response and speech and appropriateness of replies

Normal mental state (pre-morbid personality)

Varying degrees of anxiety, depression and thwarted ambition are almost universal

In the main most worries relate to home, children, marriage, work, money and sex — not necessarily in that order and usually in combination

It is invariably worthwhile discussing a patient's problems with his or her partner or close friends. The patient may be unaware of problems or their impact on other people. Furthermore, support from relatives or friends may form an invaluable component of management

say 'I feel so low (or depressed) and useless'.

Sometimes psychiatric symptoms are indicative of non-psychiatric illness. For example, depression is an invariable feature of chronic pain. Conversely, patients with psychiatric illness often present with somatic symptoms. For example, headache or abdominal pain may be the presenting feature of a depressive illness.

When taking a psychiatric history, ensure that the surroundings are comfortable and relaxing and that you are not interrupted during the story, particularly if the information is confidential.

An indication that there is a psychiatric problem either in

isolation or contributing to an underlying non-psychiatric illness usually comes during the general history and particularly when taking the social and occupational history.

Start the assessment by asking about current symptoms — 'What is wrong?' or, better, 'What are the things that are worrying you?' — and let the patient talk freely and without interruption until he or she has finished.

Patients often know what precipitated their illness, but may not reveal it immediately. 'I feel reasonable in the morning but very miserable when it gets dark, particularly if I'm on my own.' 'I get anxious and irritable whenever my husband comes into the room.'

History box 25
Questions to ask patients who have attempted suicide

Questions to ask about the overdose or other suicide attempt
What happened to make you take the overdose?
How long had you been planning it for?
Did you intend to kill yourself?
Did you expect anyone to find you?
How do you feel about it now?

Questions to ask about recent and past psychiatric history
Have you felt depressed recently?
Have you been eating well?
Have you lost any weight?
How have you been sleeping?
Have you had any previous psychiatric illnesses?
Have you ever taken an overdose before?

Questions to ask about the future
How do you see the future?
Do you have any friends or family at home or nearby?
Do you think you will take an overdose again?

Parasuicide (History box 25, above)

In hospital practice the commonest psychiatric presentation is with attempted suicide (parasuicide), which accounts for 10% of all medical admissions. Details of the time, quantity and type of overdose taken should always be sought on admission, but a full history and psychiatric assessment may not be possible because the patient is drowsy (if sedatives have been taken) or too sick and requiring emergency treatment (p. 234). Suicide notes provide useful guidance as to what the patient was thinking when they took the overdose.

As soon as possible, a careful history should be taken with the object of aiding the acute problem and preventing further attempts. About 10% of patients who take overdoses seriously intend suicide, and approximately 1% will kill themselves in the following year. Factors which increase the risk that a patient will succeed in a suicide attempt include: increasing age, male gender, living alone, recent loss (bereavement, separation from partner or redundancy), previous psychiatric history (including suicide attempts), drug or alcohol addiction, and chronic physical illness.

Ask about events leading up to the suicide attempt and what the patient expected the outcome would be. Remember that patients may often be embarrassed about their actions, and reluctant to talk at first. Ask about any recent symptoms of depression (anorexia, weight loss, insomnia) and any past psychiatric history, including depressive illness, suicide attempts or addictions. Finally, ask about how the patient sees the future and what support is available. Talk to friends or relatives if possible. Formal psychiatric referral should be made if the patient falls into the high-risk categories for succeeding in a suicide attempt, if there is evidence of psychiatric illness, if the attempt was pre-planned with the intention of eluding discovery and if there is continued suicidal intent.

SUMMARY

After taking the history summarize your findings under the headings listed in the summary box.

Once you have completed the history ask the patient whether they have any other particular worries or concerns that you have not discussed. Thank the patient and explain, if appropriate, that you would now like to proceed to examine them.

Summary box

Date and time
Place of consultation
Patient's name, age and occupation

1 Presenting complaint
Summarize both the current problem and the means by which the
patient came to medical attention
e.g. — referred by GP, with a 3-hour history of severe central chest pain
    — brought to the Accident and Emergency Department by boyfriend
after taking an overdose of paracetamol

2 History of present illness
Detailed account of current problem
If complaint is pain remember SOCRATES

3 Systematic enquiry (with detailed supplementary questions if
responses are positive)
Cardiovascular and respiratory
Gastrointestinal
Genitourinary
Gynaecological
Neurological
Musculoskeletal
Psychiatric assessment (where appropriate)

4 Past medical history
Medical:
  TB
  Hypertension
  Rheumatic fever
  Epilepsy
  Asthma
  Diabetes
Surgical
Obstetric

5 Family history
Age and state of health of parents and siblings

6 Social, occupational and travel history

7 Drug and therapy history (including allergies)

2 Examination

2

INTRODUCTION

The best way to learn how to elicit clinical signs is by demonstration and these notes are intended to supplement formal teaching in examination techniques. It is easiest to learn to examine each system separately first and then put them together to examine the 'whole' patient. A scheme is suggested on p. 147.

When examining systems remember to use, in order, the following techniques:
- inspection (look);
- palpation (feel);
- percussion (resonant = hollow, dull = solid);
- auscultation (listen).

When examining the abdomen, abnormal joints or any obviously inflamed site:
- always ask the patient if there is any pain present;
- always examine painful areas with tenderness;
- never examine beyond the pain threshold.

You may find it helpful to practise examination techniques on a friend before examining patients.

Physical examination begins before taking the history by observing the patient as they walk, sit and stand. Pay particular attention to the face, posture and gait. There is a typical facial appearance in a number of common disorders (Examination box 1, p. 53).

To help get started at the bedside, summaries of what to look for and examine are given in Examination boxes 1–9. Fuller descriptions are given in the text.

Everyone finds examining patients difficult when first on the wards, until the techniques become familiar through practice.

HANDS AND NAILS

Hand signs

To avoid causing unnecessary pain, ask 'Is there any pain in your arms or joints?' before taking hold of the patient's hand to examine it. Holding the patient's hand is also a further way of gaining their confidence.

Examination box 1
First impressions

Facial appearance

Pain	Is the patient in obvious pain?
Obesity	Is the patient overweight?
Severe anaemia	Pallor
Hypothyroidism	Periorbital puffiness
	Dry skin
	Coarse hair
Hyperthyroidism	Prominent staring eyes of exophthalmos
Facial palsy	Drooping of one side of the face
Parkinson's disease	Blank, expressionless face

Posture

Causes of stooping or slouching	Normal in the elderly
	Pain
	Depression
	Spinal deformity (less common)
	Collapsed vertebra due to osteoporosis, ankylosing spondylitis in young men

Gait	See p. 129

Examine the hand for moist palms, clubbing, palmar erythema, spider naevi, splinter haemorrhages, Dupuytren's contracture and joint swelling and deformities.

Moist palms

Causes Moist palms suggest anxiety (hands often cool) or thyrotoxicosis (hands usually warm).

Palmar erythema

Examination Palmar erythema means red palms.

Causes It occurs in pregnancy, thyrotoxicosis, chronic liver disease and rheumatoid arthritis, but also some in normal people.

Spider naevi

Examination Spider naevi are dilated small blood vessels which blanch when the central feeding arteriole (the body of the spider) is pressed, and then refill. They are distributed in the area drained by the superior vena cava.

Causes Spider naevi are associated with high circulating oestrogen levels and are a feature of alcoholic and chronic liver disease (reduced liver metabolism) and pregnancy. A small number (less than five) may be found in normal people.

Osler's nodes

Examination Osler's nodes are painful, red, infarcts in the fingertips.

Cause They are a feature of infective endocarditis. They are exceedingly rare.

Dupuytren's contracture

Examination Dupuytren's contracture is fibrosis of the palmar fascia which causes flexion deformities of one or more fingers. The thickened fascia can invariably be seen and always felt.

Causes It often occurs in manual workers following repeated trauma to the palm of the hand, and is associated with chronic liver disease. It has a familial tendency.

Hand joints (Fig. 2.1)

Examination Ask about pain and look for swelling or deformity.

Causes Painful, swollen or deformed hand joints are usually due to osteo-, rheumatoid or gouty arthritis. In osteoarthritis the terminal finger joints are commonly affected, whereas in rheumatoid arthritis symmetrical involvement of the proximal joints gives rise to the characteristic swan neck or boutonnière deformities. Gouty arthritis is usually asymmetrical, affecting one or more joints. The joint is usually red, warm, swollen and exquisitely tender. White deposits of uric acid crystals (tophi) may be visible in or around the joint.

Heberden's nodes are bony nodules at the terminal finger joints which occur in osteoarthritis.

Nail changes (Fig. 2.2)

Clubbing

Examination Clubbing begins as sponginess of the nailbed due

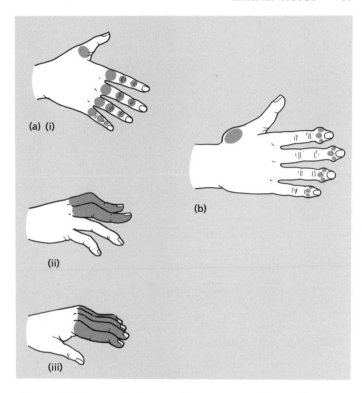

Fig. 2.1 (a) Rheumatoid arthritis. (i) Proximal interphalangeal involvement with ulnar deviation of the fingers; (ii) boutonnière deformity; (iii) swan neck deformity. (b) Osteoarthritis. Involvement of distal interphalangeal joints with Heberden's nodes and the first metacarpal joint of the thumb.

to fluid deposition, which progresses so that the normal angle of the nailbed is lost. In advanced cases, the terminal phalanx swells, giving the fingers a 'drumstick' appearance.

Causes

• Certain pulmonary diseases, including malignancy (carcinoma, mesothelioma), chronic suppurative disease (abscess, empyema, bronchiectasis, cystic fibrosis, tuberculosis (TB)) and fibrosing alveolitis;

2

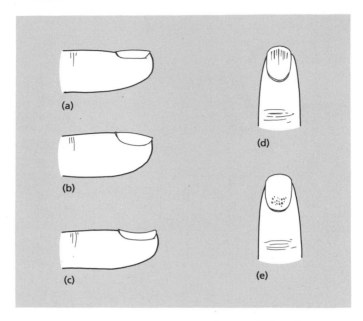

Fig. 2.2 Nail changes. (a) Normal; (b) clubbing; (c) koilonychia; (d) splinter haemorrhages; (e) nail pitting.

- certain types of heart disease (cyanotic heart disease and infective endocarditis);
- certain types of abdominal disease (inflammatory bowel disease, cirrhosis).

Splinter haemorrhages

Examination Splinter haemorrhages are longitudinal linear haemorrhages under the nails.

Causes Splinter haemorrhages in nails are often traumatic. They also occur in infective endocarditis, as the result of micro-emboli from the infected valve or an associated vasculitis.

Other nail changes

Leukonychia (white nails) is associated with hypoproteinaemia (liver disease, nephrotic syndrome). Koilonychia (concave, spoon-shaped nails) occurs in iron deficiency. Pitting of the nails (numerous small, pin-sized holes) is a feature of psoriasis. Fungal infection causes thickening and destruction of the nails.

Cyanosis

Examination Cyanosis refers to blue discoloration of the nail-beds, lips and tongue. It results from the presence of reduced haemoglobin (more than 3 g/100 ml) due to arterial hypoxaemia. Thus an anaemic patient with severe hypoxaemia may not be cyanosed. Patients with methaemoglobinaemia may be cyanosed (look blue) but not be hypoxic, and patients with carboxyhaemoglobinaemia look pink but are nevertheless hypoxic.

Causes Cyanosis may be:
- peripheral — due to poor circulation;
- central — due either to pulmonary disease that reduces alveolar oxygen transport or to cyanotic heart disease when blood passes directly from the right to the left side of the heart through a congenital defect without passing through the lungs. In central cyanosis the tongue is always blue.

HEAD AND NECK EXAMINATION

Head

Facial expression

Examination Look at the patient's face.

Causes of reduced or absent facial expression: depression and Parkinson's disease.

Skin

Examination Look for skin rashes or spider naevi (see p. 53).

Eyes (Fig. 2.3)

Periorbital swelling

Examination Oedema readily collects in the soft lax tissues around the eyes.

Causes Periorbital swelling is common in association with

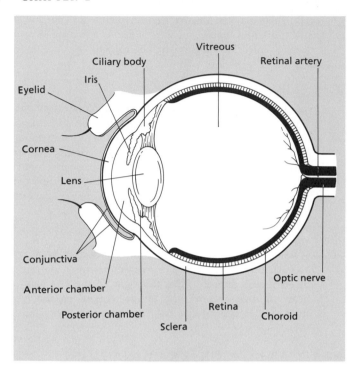

Fig. 2.3 Anatomy of the eye.

local irritation and, less commonly, with hypothyroidism (myxoedema), as a result of the deposition of mucopolysaccharides, and the nephrotic syndrome.

Lid retraction

Examination Lid retraction means that the sclera is visible between the upper eyelid and the iris. It may be accompanied by a tendency for the eyelid to 'lag' behind the iris when the patient is asked to look down quickly by following a moving finger, whilst the head is kept still.

Causes Lid retraction occurs in both anxiety and hyperthyroidism, whereas the presence of lid lag usually indicates hyperthyroidism.

Exophthalmos

Examination Exophthalmos means that the eyeball is prominent and the sclera is visible above the lower eyelid.

Cause It occurs in Graves' disease (hyperthyroidism due to autoimmune thyroiditis) as a result of swelling of the retro-orbital tissues.

Conjunctivae

Examination The conjunctiva, which covers the whole of the front of the eye (pupil, iris, sclera and inner part of the eyelid) is normally translucent.

Causes of abnormalities Pallor of the conjunctival mucous membrane is an inaccurate clinical indicator of anaemia, while yellowness of the sclera is often the earliest sign of jaundice.

Conjunctivitis is usually due to infection or a foreign body.

Subconjunctival haemorrhages often have no obvious cause but may indicate an underlying bleeding disorder or follow excessive coughing or minor trauma.

Mouth

Herpes labialis (cold sores)

Examination Herpes labialis is characterized by the formation of irritable vesicles (small fluid-filled blisters), which scab. The lesions are common and often recurrent.

Causes Herpes labialis infection is caused by herpes simplex virus. Rarely it indicates underlying infection (particularly pneumonia) or immunodeficiency (e.g. acquired immuno-deficiency syndrome (AIDS)).

Stomatitis

Examination Angular stomatitis is characterized by inflamed cracks at the corners of the mouth. Ulceration may also occur inside the mouth.

Causes Stomatitis usually indicates old ill-fitting dentures, but is also a feature of iron and vitamin B deficiencies. Mouth ulcers may be due to infection (commonly *Candida albicans* (thrush) or Coxsackie A virus), due to recurrent aphthous ulceration or associated with inflammatory bowel disease or coeliac disease.

Tongue

Examination Examine the upper and lower surfaces of the tongue held both inside and out of the mouth.

Causes of abnormalities Pallor of the tongue is a poor indicator of anaemia, but dryness of the tongue is a useful indicator of dehydration. Dryness is also a feature of mouth breathing.

Blueness of the tongue indicates central cyanosis.

A smooth tongue (atrophic glossitis) results from iron, vitamin B_{12} and folate deficiencies, as well as from treatment with antibiotics. The condition is often painful.

White patches on a sore red tongue are usually due to fungal infection with *Candida albicans* (thrush).

Teeth and gums

Examination The state of hygiene of teeth and gums should always be noted as they are a common source of infection.

Causes of gum hypertrophy Usually drug therapy, most commonly with the anti-epileptic phenytoin or the immuno-suppressive drug cyclosporin A.

Neck (Fig. 2.4)

Examination Before testing any movements ask: 'Is the neck painful to move?' to avoid causing pain.

The neck should be examined from the front and from behind. Inspect for lumps, scars and pulsations, both arterial and venous (see p. 67). Then palpate the neck:

• feel from the front for abnormal masses and lymph nodes along the muscles bordering the posterior triangle (sternomastoid and trapezius), and along the suboccipital and supraclavicular chains;

• ask the patient to sit forward, and feel the front of the neck from behind for lymph nodes and masses, particularly of the thyroid and salivary glands.

Thyroid

Examination Enlargement of the thyroid (goitre) causes swelling around the thyroid cartilage. It may extend into the superior mediastinum so that you cannot feel a lower border. If the

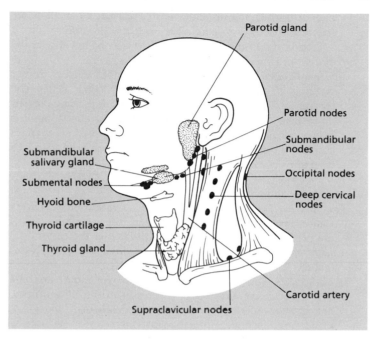

Fig. 2.4 Anatomy of the neck.

goitre is entirely retrosternal you will not be able to palpate it in the neck.

The thyroid moves up and down on swallowing and should be inspected and palpated whilst the patient drinks a glass of water. Note the consistency and any tenderness of the gland, and look for associated features of:

• hyperthyroidism — warm moist skin, tremor, fast pressurized voice, tachycardia, atrial fibrillation, tachyarrhythmia exophthalmos, conjunctivitis, lid retraction, lid lag, diplopia, hyperactivity, irritability, nervousness;

• hypothyroidism — dry, coarse, sparse hair, slow voice, bradycardia, periorbital puffiness, intellectual impairment, deafness.

Retrosternal goitres can cause compression of the oesophagus or trachea and difficulty with breathing or swallowing, and cause dullness to percussion over the sternum.

A bruit due to increased blood flow may be heard over the thyroid in hyperthyroidism.

Causes of goitre Causes include puberty (which causes a diffuse swelling of the gland), hypothyroidism (iodine deficiency, Hashimoto's thyroiditis), Graves' disease (autoimmune hyperthyroidism), benign cysts and carcinoma. Rarely, thyroiditis may occur as part of a viral infection (De Quervain's thyroiditis) or as part of a chronic fibrotic process (Reidel's thyroiditis).

Submandibular and parotid glands

Examination Feel for swelling of the submandibular salivary glands, just inside the inner border of the mandible, and of the parotid glands, just below and in front of the ears.

Causes of submandibular and parotid gland swelling Causes include:
- infection — usually mumps, but also from mouth bacteria (streptococci and anaerobes), especially in the ill and dehydrated, and in patients with ill-fitting dentures;
- tumours — benign and malignant;
- generalized inflammatory processes such as sarcoidosis (see pp. 161–2).

CARDIOVASCULAR EXAMINATION
(Examination box 2, p. 63)

Hands

Examine the hands for:
- cyanosis (central due to hypoxia in cardiac failure or left-to-right shunts, peripheral due to poor peripheral circulation or vasoconstriction in cardiac failure);
- clubbing (subacute bacterial endocarditis, cyanotic heart disease);
- splinter haemorrhages, Osler's nodes (bacterial endocarditis);
- moist palms (thyrotoxicosis, anxiety).

Examination box 2
Cardiovascular system (see pp. 62–78)

Hands	Look for clubbing, peripheral cyanosis, splinter haemorrhages, Osler's nodes
Mouth	Look for central cyanosis
Pulse	Measure its rate, rhythm and character, using the brachial pulse. Palpate all peripheral pulses, comparing both radials, and radial and femoral on one side (for radiofemoral delay). Auscultate over carotids, above umbilicus (i.e. over renal arteries) and over femorals for bruits
Blood pressure	Look for high (higher than 140/90 mmHg) or low blood pressure (less than 90 mmHg systolic). It varies with age. Note whether the pulse pressure is widened (e.g. 190/60), as occurs in aortic regurgitation, or narrowed (e.g. 100/70), as occurs in aortic stenosis
Conjunctivae	Look for severe anaemia
Tongue and lips	Look for central cyanosis
Jugular venous pulse (JVP)	Note any elevation. Note any 'a' (corresponds with atrial systole) or 'v' (ventricular systole) wave prominence
Apex beat	Feel for left ventricular hypertrophy at the anatomical apex. Feel for right ventricular hypertrophy (indicated by a left parasternal heave). (Percussion of the heart for size is valueless)
Thrills	Feel for thrills, which indicate underlying murmurs (or rarely pericarditis)
Heart sounds	Listen to the heart
Abdomen	Feel for enlarged liver (right heart failure; pulsatile in tricuspid regurgitation)
Legs	Look for oedema (right heart failure), evidence of deep vein thrombosis (DVT) or peripheral vascular disease

2

Pulse

Pulse rate and rhythm

Examination Feel the radial pulse to assess its rate and note any irregularity.

Causes of abnormalities Complete irregularity (irregularly irregular pulse) occurs in atrial fibrillation. Occasional irregular beats are usually due to extra beats (extrasystoles), which can often be eliminated by exercise.

The common pulse abnormalities are:

- sinus tachycardia (exercise, thyrotoxicosis, anxiety);
- sinus bradycardia (athletes, myxoedema, hypothermia, beta-blocking drugs);
- atrial fibrillation (untreated ventricular rate usually 110–150).

Other common arrhythmias are:

- paroxysmal atrial tachycardia (untreated ventricular rate usually 160–200);
- atrial flutter (untreated ventricular rate usually 100–150);
- ventricular tachycardia.

These can be distinguished only on the electrocardiogram (ECG) (p. 294).

- Ventricular fibrillation is associated with no cardiac output leading to cardiac arrest (p. 305).

Pulse character

Pulse character is difficult to assess — use the brachial or carotid pulses. Pulse pressure is best determined by measuring the blood pressure.

Collapsing pulse

Examination A collapsing pulse is characterized by a rapid rise and fall.

Causes It indicates aortic regurgitation or an increased cardiac output, which may be due to anaemia, pregnancy, thyrotoxicosis or an arteriovenous fistula.

Plateau pulse

Examination A plateau pulse has a slow rise and fall.

Cause It occurs in aortic stenosis.

Pulsus paradoxus

Examination Pulsus paradoxus is accentuation of the normal decrease in amplitude of the arterial pulse during inspiration. In normal people this probably occurs because the capacity of the pulmonary vascular bed increases during inspiration, reducing the return of blood to the left ventricle. This is partly compensated for by an increased right ventricular output in inspiration.

Causes Pulsus paradoxus may indicate obstructive airways disease (asthma and chronic bronchitis), pericardial constriction or right ventricular failure:

• in obstructive airways disease the powerful inspiratory effort reduces intrathoracic pressure more than normal and therefore increases the capacity of the lung vessels;

• in pericardial constriction or right ventricular failure the right ventricle is unable to compensate for the increased pulmonary vascular capacity by increasing its output.

Arterial pulses

Examination Confirm the presence of the radial, brachial, carotid, superficial temporal, femoral, popliteal, dorsalis pedis and posterior tibial pulses on both right and left sides. Palpate both radial pulses together (feeling for differences in pulse volume between the two sides), and the right radial pulse at the same time as the right femoral pulse (feeling for a delay in the onset of the femoral pulse — radiofemoral delay).

Listen to the carotid and femoral pulses with a stethoscope as partial occlusion may cause turbulent flow, which is audible as a bruit.

Look for evidence of chronic ischaemia in the legs as indicated by the following:

• absent pulses;
• cold feet;
• dry skin and lack of hair;
• ulceration or gangrene.

Causes of abnormal findings Absence of an arterial pulse usually indicates arterial narrowing or occlusion due to atheroma, or an embolus. Radiofemoral delay is a feature of coarctation of the aorta (p. 76). Asymmetry between the radial pulses may be due to congenital absence of the pulse, arterial narrowing or occlusion on one side or coarctation of the aorta.

If aortic coarctation is suspected the blood pressure should be measured in both arms.

Blood pressure

Technique

Blood pressure is measured using a sphygmomanometer and the brachial artery. When taking blood pressure check that the cuff of the sphygmomanometer is an appropriate size (70–80% of the arm circumference should be covered with the bladder of the cuff) – a large cuff is needed for very large arms.

The cuff is inflated around the upper arm until the brachial pulse cannot be felt. The pressure is then slowly released (allow the mercury column to fall 2–3 mmHg/second) whilst listening over the brachial artery.

Korotkoff sounds

Examination Korotkoff described five sounds. The first sound occurs as the cuff pressure is released and blood begins to flow through the brachial artery, and corresponds with the systolic blood pressure. Turbulence of the blood flow may then cause the sound:

- to fade (sound 2);
- and then increase (sound 3);
- before finally muffling (sound 4);
- and disappearing (sound 5).

Sounds 2 and 3 are of no clinical relevance and should be ignored.

It is conventional that the fifth sound is taken as the diastolic pressure (use the fourth sound if the fifth is inaudible – e.g. in pregnancy or in hyperkinetic states). The position of the patient whilst the blood pressure is taken (lying, sitting or standing) and the arm (left or right) should be recorded.

If pulsus paradoxus is suspected, its presence can be more accurately assessed whilst measuring the blood pressure. The pressure in the cuff is slowly released, and in pulsus paradoxus only the stronger pulsations will be heard at first because the pulse volume varies with respiration. As the pressure in the cuff is released further, all of the pulsations become audible. The difference (in mmHg) between hearing the first sounds and hearing all of the sounds is a direct measure of the paradox.

Jugular venous pulse (JVP) (Fig. 2.5, p. 68)

The jugular veins communicate directly with the right atrium and are therefore a useful manometer for measuring right atrial (or 'central venous') pressure (normal: 2–5 cm).

Examination With the patient lying at an angle of 45° and with adequate (preferably oblique) lighting, identify the internal jugular vein, which runs from the ear lobe to the medial end of the clavicle, between the heads of sternomastoid. Venous pulsation should be just visible above the clavicle, at a level corresponding with the sternal angle, which is usually taken as the reference point for estimating central venous pressure (CVP).

The external jugular vein, running from the angle of the jaw to the mid-point of the clavicle, is often easier to see than the internal jugular vein, but may give a less reliable measurement if trapped in superficial tissues.

Venous pulsation can be distinguished from arterial pulsation because:
• it has a complex waveform (see below);
• it is impalpable;
• it can be abolished if venous emptying is obstructed by pressure over the root of the neck;
• it can be pushed up by gentle pressure over the upper abdomen (hepatojugular reflex) or by the Valsalva manoeuvre (forced expiration against a closed glottis).

Changes in the right atrial pressure during the cardiac cycle cause three characteristic positive waves in the venous pulsations:
• the 'a' (atrial contraction) wave coincides with atrial contraction, and is followed by the 'x' descent;
• a small 'c' wave interrupts the 'x' descent at the onset of ventricular systole and is caused by carotid pulsation;
• the 'v' (ventricular contraction) wave occurs as the right

2

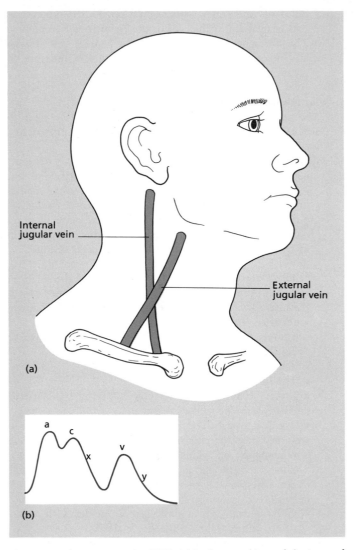

Fig. 2.5 Jugular venous pulse (JVP). (a) Surface markings of the internal and external jugular veins; (b) JVP waveform.

atrium refills and the tricuspid valve is closed, and is followed by the 'y' descent as the tricuspid valve reopens.

In practice only the 'a' and 'v' waves are visible.

Causes of increased JVP An increase in the height of the JVP reflects either an increase in right atrial pressure or obstruction in the root of the neck — superior vena caval (SVC) obstruction.

Increased right atrial pressure is usually due to failure of the heart to pump blood through the circulation adequately. It may be accompanied by distension of the liver and oedema around the ankles.

In SVC obstruction the JVP is fixed and has no waveform.

JVP *waveform* is *abnormal* if there is abnormal emptying or filling of the right side of the heart, as a result of either structural or rhythm abnormalities as follows:

• The 'a' wave becomes prominent if there is resistance to emptying of the right atrium, as in tricuspid stenosis, pulmonary valve stenosis or pulmonary hypertension.

• The 'a' wave is absent in atrial fibrillation because there is no coordinated atrial contraction.

• The 'v' wave becomes prominent in tricuspid regurgitation.

• A prominent 'cannon' wave is a large 'a' wave and occurs when the right atrium contracts against a closed triscuspid valve because the atria and ventricles are contracting at the same time. This occurs with every beat if the stimulus for contraction arises in the atrioventricular (AV) node rather than the sinoatrial (SA) node (nodal rhythm) and at intervals in complete heart block.

• The 'x' descent tends to disappear in atrial fibrillation because it is mostly due to atrial diastole, but this is not an easily detectable or particularly useful sign.

• A steep 'y' descent (diastolic collapse) occurs in constrictive pericarditis, when the venous pressure is kept high during the rest of the cardiac cycle.

Heart (Fig. 2.6)

Cardiac apex

Examination Feel for the cardiac apex, which is the lowermost and outermost point at which the impulse of the heart can be felt. Normally it is within the mid-clavicular line and not below the fifth rib space.

Causes of abnormal findings Displacement outward and downward of the cardiac apex indicates either enlargement of the heart or mediastinal shift.

The mediastinum may be 'pushed' across the chest cavity when there is air or fluid in the pleural space (i.e. a pneumothorax or a pleural effusion) on the other side, or 'pulled' across by collapse of the lung on the same side.

A prominent or thrusting apex beat usually indicates left

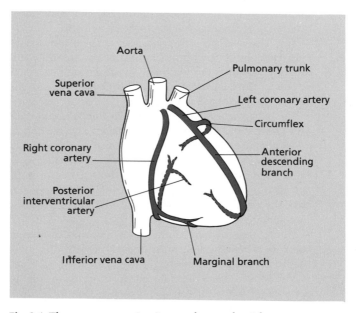

Fig. 2.6 The coronary arteries. In most hearts, the right coronary artery supplies the sinus node, the AV node and bundle, the right ventricle and the inferior part of the left ventricle. The left coronary artery divides into the anterior descending branch, which supplies the interventricular septum and the anterior wall of the left ventricle, and the circumflex, which supplies the lateral and posterior aspects of the left ventricle.

ventricular hypertrophy. In contrast, right ventricular hypertrophy causes a prominent lift to the left of the sternum (left parasternal heave).

The cardiac apex may be impalpable if the patient is fat or if there is fluid in the pleural or pericardial space (i.e. something between the heart apex and the examining hand). It may become easier to feel by asking the patient to lie on his/her left side.

Thrills

Examination Feel for thrills over the valves (Fig. 2.7, p. 72). Thrills are felt as vibrations and are usually caused by abnormal eddy currents of blood around abnormal heart valves.

Heart sounds

Examination Learning to recognize abnormalities of the heart sounds can be achieved only by listening to as many normal and abnormal hearts as possible. Establish and become familiar with a pattern of listening that you find comfortable. *NB*: A suggested stethoscopic route and diagrammatic representations of abnormalities that may be heard are given in Fig. 2.7.

The first heart sound corresponds to closure of the mitral and tricuspid valves in that order, and corresponds to ventricular systole and the carotid artery pulsation in the neck. The second heart sound is caused by closure of the aortic and pulmonary valves. It may be 'split' (audible as two separate sounds) on inspiration (physiological splitting), or with right bundle branch block or atrial septal defect, all of which delay emptying of the right ventricle. Reverse splitting (pulmonary valve closes before aortic valve) occurs with left bundle branch block. A third heart sound may be heard just after the second sound (ventricular filling). It is common in young people, but should be regarded as abnormal after the age of 40, when it implies right or left ventricular disease. The fourth heart sound occurs just before the first sound (atrial systole). It is associated with 'ventricular stiffness' due to hypertension, aortic stenosis or myocardial infarction.

AORTIC VALVE (A)

Stenosis

③ Right 2nd intercostal space

Soft A₂

Ejection systolic

Regurgitation

② Lower left sternal edge

Early diastolic

PULMONARY (P)

④ Left 2nd intercostal space

Stenosis

Soft P₂

Ejection systolic

Regurgitation

Early diastolic

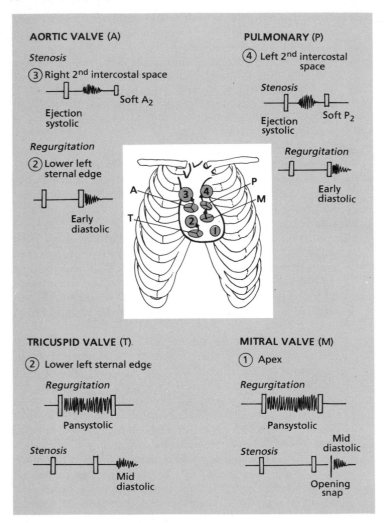

TRICUSPID VALVE (T)

② Lower left sternal edge

Regurgitation

Pansystolic

Stenosis

Mid diastolic

MITRAL VALVE (M)

① Apex

Regurgitation

Pansystolic

Stenosis

Mid diastolic

Opening snap

Fig. 2.7 Suggested stethoscopic route (1–4) for listening to heart valves. 1, Apex; 2, lower left sternal edge; 3, right second intercostal space; 4, left second intercostal space. → = direction of blood flow.

Murmurs

Examination Use the bell of the stethoscope for low-pitched sounds, particularly those of mitral stenosis, and the diaphragm for high-pitched sounds, i.e. those of aortic or pulmonary regurgitation.

To enhance murmurs make sure that you:

• turn a patient onto the left side when listening to the mitral valve;

• sit them forward holding their breath in expiration (reduces airspace between heart and stethoscope), while you listen to the aortic valve.

The features of the commonly heard murmurs are shown in Fig. 2.7.

Clinical findings in valve lesions and congenital cardiac defects are as follows below.

Aortic stenosis

Pulse Rhythm — usually sinus (atrial fibrillation suggests coexisting mitral valve disease). Plateau pulse — reduced volume, slow rise and fall.

Blood pressure Normal or reduced pulse pressure (hypertension with small pulse pressure may occur).

JVP Normal (unless accompanied by heart failure).

Palpation Apex may be 'heaving' due to left ventricular hypertrophy.

Auscultation Loud, harsh mid-systolic ejection murmur; best heard in second left intercostal space (sometimes loudest at apex); often radiates to carotids; may be accompanied by a systolic ejection click (disappears if valve is immobile due to heavy calcification).

Aortic regurgitation

Pulse Rhythm — usually sinus. Large-volume collapsing pulse; may be visible pulsation of carotids (Corrigan's sign).

Blood pressure Wide pulse pressure.

JVP Normal (unless accompanied by heart failure).

Palpation Apex displaced and heaving (dilated, hypertrophied left ventricle).

Auscultation Blowing, high-pitched early diastolic murmur; loudest in third and fourth left intercostal space — sit patient forward, holding breath in expiration, and listen with diaphragm.

Mitral stenosis

Pulse Rhythm — atrial fibrillation common. Small volume (due to reduced cardiac output).

Blood pressure Normal or low (reduced cardiac output).

JVP Normal (unless accompanied by heart failure).

Palpation Position of apex usually normal; may be 'palpable' first sound, felt as a tapping impulse before the ventricular impulse.

Auscultation Loud first sound (unless valve mobility reduced by calcification); opening snap (high-pitched early diastolic sound); mid-diastolic murmur — long, low frequency (listen with bell); rumbling murmur, best heard at the apex with patient rolled to left side.

Mitral regurgitation

Pulse Rhythm — usually sinus; atrial fibrillation may occur.

Blood pressure Usually normal.

JVP Normal (unless accompanied by heart failure).

Palpation Apex diffuse and thrusting, displaced laterally.

Auscultation Apical pansystolic murmur radiating to the axilla.

Tricuspid regurgitation

Pulse Rhythm — invariably atrial fibrillation.

JVP Raised with prominent systolic wave.

Palpation Prominent right ventricular impulse ('heave') at left sternal edge.

Auscultation Pansystolic murmur may be (but is not always) heard at lower left sternal edge, loudest on inspiration.

Other findings Pulsatile, enlarged liver; ascites; oedema.

Tricuspid stenosis (rare)

Pulse Rhythm — usually atrial fibrillation; low volume (low cardiac output).

JVP Prominent 'a' wave if sinus rhythm.

Auscultation Rumbling mid-diastolic murmur best heard at the left lower sternal edge; louder on inspiration.

Pulmonary stenosis (rare)

Pulse Low volume.

JVP Large 'a' wave.

Palpation Prominent right ventricular impulse ('heave') at left sternal edge.

Auscultation Harsh mid-systolic ejection murmur, best heard on inspiration in second left intercostal space.

Pulmonary regurgitation

This is usually due to a dilated pulmonary valve ring caused by pulmonary hypertension.

Auscultation Early diastolic murmur, maximal in second and third left intercostal spaces.

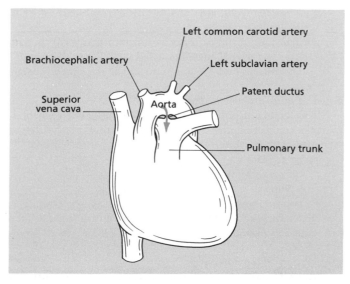

Fig. 2.8 Patent ductus arteriosus.

Atrial septal defect (ASD)

Pulse Normal or atrial fibrillation.

Blood pressure Usually normal.

JVP Usually normal.

Palpation May be left parasternal heave of right ventricular hypertrophy.

Auscultation Wide, fixed splitting of second sound. Flow through the defect (which is wide with a low pressure gradient) does not cause a murmur, but increased flow through the right side of the heart may cause a pulmonary diastolic murmur or a tricuspid systolic murmur.

Ventricular septal defect (VSD)

Signs depend on size of shunt; a small defect ('maladie de Roger') may give rise to a loud murmur but no other abnormal cardiovascular findings. A large defect with shunting of large volumes of blood through the lungs may cause pulmonary hypertension.

Pulse, blood pressure and JVP Usually normal.

Palpation Forceful apex and left parasternal heave if right ventricular hypertrophy.

Auscultation Loud pansystolic murmur and thrill, maximal at lower left sternal edge. Increased flow across the mitral valve may cause a mid-diastolic murmur if the shunt is large.

Patent ductus arteriosus (Fig. 2.8, p. 75)

The ductus arteriosus, derived from the sixth branchial arch and connecting the left pulmonary artery to the descending aorta, fails to close.

Pulse Collapsing.

Blood pressure Wide volume.

JVP Normal.

Palpation Prominent apex (left ventricular hypertrophy).

Auscultation Continuous 'machinery' murmur maximal under the left clavicle.

Coarctation of the aorta (Fig. 2.9)

In 98% of patients, narrowing of the aorta occurs just distal to the origin of the left subclavian artery. A collateral arterial

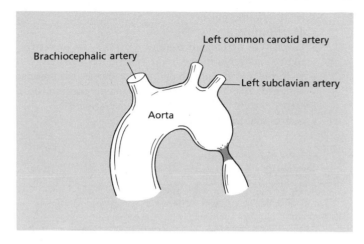

Fig. 2.9 Coarctation of the aorta (distal to the origin of the left subclavian artery in 98% of cases).

circulation develops in the periscapular and intercostal arteries.

Pulse and blood pressure Hypertension in the upper limbs and weak, delayed pulses in the legs (radiofemoral delay).

Palpation Prominent apex of left ventricular hypertrophy may be present.

Auscultation Systolic murmur at front and back of the left upper thorax. Murmurs from the collateral circulation may be heard over the scapulae.

Fallot's tetralogy

VSD, pulmonary stenosis, right ventricular hypertrophy and overriding aorta (aorta is positioned over the VSD).

Signs Cyanosis, clubbing; left parasternal heave of right ventricular hypertrophy; mid-systolic murmur of pulmonary stenosis (there is no murmur from the large VSD).

Pulmonary hypertension

Signs

• Malar flush — cyanosis or dusky pink discoloration of upper cheeks;

- small-volume pulse;
- atrial fibrillation;
- raised JVP — tricuspid regurgitation may be present;
- right parasternal heave (right ventricular hypertrophy);
- 'palpable' pulmonary component of the second heart sound;
- enlarged liver — pulsatile if tricuspid regurgitation also present;
- ascites and peripheral oedema.

Examination box 3
Respiratory system

Hands	Look for clubbing and peripheral cyanosis
Conjunctivae	Look for severe anaemia
Mouth	Look for central cyanosis
Neck	Feel for cervical lymphadenopathy, which may be secondary to bronchial carcinoma. Look for a raised JVP, which suggests superior vena caval obstruction or right heart strain from chronic obstructive airways disease. Note whether the trachea is central or displaced
Front of the chest	Observe chest movements for symmetry and expansion. Note any scars. Palpate for thrills. Percuss and note any dullness. Auscultate for breath sounds
Back of the chest	Sit the patient forward and feel their neck for glands, which are most easily felt from behind. Observe chest movements for symmetry and expansion. Note any scars. Palpate for thrills. Percuss, noting any dullness. Auscultate for breath sounds

---

EXAMINATION OF THE RESPIRATORY SYSTEM (Examination box 3, above, and Table 2.1, pp. 80−1)

It is best to examine the anterior chest completely before examining the back so that the patient has to move only once.

Using the system of inspection, palpation, percussion and auscultation, most chest problems can be accurately defined.

Respiratory rate

Examination The respiratory rate should preferably be measured without the patient being aware, so that they do not try and control it themselves. Pretend to be measuring the pulse. Count the number of respirations taken by the patient during 1 minute.

Causes of abnormal respiratory rate An increase in the respiratory rate above the normal 12–16 breaths per minute and the use of accessory respiratory muscles in the neck usually indicates respiratory disease. Metabolic acidosis of renal failure and diabetic ketoacidosis also increase respiratory rate.

Appearance of chest wall

Examination Look for any scars or deformities of the chest wall such as anterior or lateral bending of the spine (kyphosis or scoliosis respectively). A barrel-shaped chest may result from overinflation of the lungs in airways obstruction.

Trachea

Examination Feel the position of the trachea in the suprasternal notch with the neck extended to bring the trachea forward. The trachea is best felt by placing the ring and index fingers on the sternoclavicular joints and gently rolling the middle finger forward over the suprasternal notch.

Causes of deviation Deviation to one side may be due to local pressure from a goitre or a tumour, spinal curvature or shift of the upper mediastinum. The trachea is 'pulled' towards fibrosis of an upper lobe and 'pushed' away from a large pleural effusion or pneumothorax.

Chest expansion

Examination Some idea of the range of movements of the two sides of the chest may be gained by inspection, but this is more accurately assessed by palpation. Gently grasp the patient's chest around the lower rib cage with outstretched hands so that the tips of the thumbs meet in the mid-line and ask the patient to take a deep breath. The movement of the thumbs away from the mid-line is a measure of the chest expansion on each side. Check upper chest expansion as well, with the hands flat on the chest below the clavicles.

Causes of reduced expansion Reduced expansion on one side is

Table 2.1 Physical signs in lung disease

	Chest wall movement	Tracheal displacement	Percussion note	Breath sounds	Tactile vocal resonance and fremitus
Consolidation:	Reduced on side of lesion	None (unless associated collapse)	Dull	Bronchial	Increased
Collapse:	Reduced on side of lesion	Towards side of lesion if upper lobe	Dull	Reduced (may be bronchial)	Reduced
Fibrosis:	Reduced on side of lesion	Towards side of lesion if upper lobe/apex	Dull	Bronchial	Increased
Pleural effusion:	Reduced on side of lesion	Central (may deviate away from large effusion)	Stony dull	Reduced (may be bronchial at top of effusion)	Reduced

Pneumothorax:	Reduced on side of lesion	Usually central (may deviate away if large)	Normal or hyper-resonant	Reduced	Reduced
Asthma:	Symmetrical reduction	None	Normal	Reduced with wheeze	Normal
Pulmonary oedema:	Normal	None	Normal	Normal with fine inspiratory crackles	Normal

Helpful tips: decreased movement on one side of the chest means that there is disease in the underlying lung on that side. All the special signs (i.e. bronchial breathing, tactile fremitus, vocal resonance and whispering pectoriloquy) occur only in consolidation and the much rarer fibrosis.

caused by underlying lung disease on the same side – e.g. pleural effusion, pneumothorax, consolidation, collapse and fibrosis.

There is symmetrical reduction of chest expansion in airways obstruction.

Percussion

Percussion distinguishes resonant, hollow or air-filled spaces such as lung from dull, solid organs such as the liver or fluid-filled spaces such as a pleural effusion.

Technique Place the left middle finger firmly over the area to be percussed and strike it with the tip of the right middle finger.

The technique and the characteristic sound and feel of resonant and dull spaces can only be mastered and recognized by practice.

Start by percussing over the clavicles and then move down the chest, comparing the percussion note on the left and right side in turn. Do not forget the apices or the lateral aspects.

The surface markings of the lungs are shown in Fig. 2.10 on p. 83. The upper border of the liver, which is dull to percussion, is the fourth right intercostal space, which is the nipple line in men.

Causes of abnormalities Dullness to percussion is caused by:
- pleural thickening;
- pleural effusion, which produces a stony dullness;
- pulmonary fibrosis;
- consolidation;
- collapse.

Hyperresonance is a feature of pneumothorax (air-filled space between the chest wall and a collapsed lung).

Auscultation

The character and intensity of the breath sounds and the presence of any added sounds are assessed by auscultation.

Technique Ask the patient to breathe in and out deeply and slowly through their mouth. Listen first over the apices above the clavicles and work systematically downwards at 5 cm (1.5–2 in.) intervals, comparing left and right side in turn.

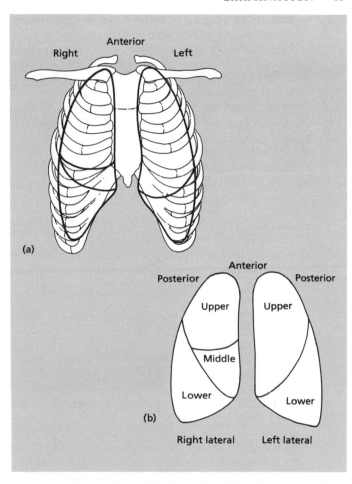

Fig. 2.10 Surface markings of the lungs. (a) Oblique fissures run along the line of fifth/sixth rib. Horizontal fissure runs from fourth costal cartilage to sixth rib in mid-axillary line. (b) Note: posteriorly you are listening mainly to lower lobes. Anteriorly you are listening mainly to upper lobes and on the right the middle lobe.

Examination Breath sounds are produced by the passage of air through the upper respiratory tract. They are therefore loudest over the trachea and upper airways where they are heard as a harsh, blowing inspiratory sound followed after a pause by an expiratory sound of similar character. These sounds are called bronchial breath sounds.

Breath sounds are modified by transmission through the smaller airways and are heard over the rest of the chest as a lower-pitched sound throughout inspiration followed immediately by a shorter expiratory sound. These are normal vesicular breath sounds.

Causes of bronchial breath sounds Transmission of bronchial breath sounds to the chest wall is favoured by:
- consolidation (pneumonia);
- fibrosis;
- cavitation.

Bronchial breathing will be heard over the affected areas.

Causes of diminished-intensity breath sounds Due to impaired transmission and include:
- collapse of a lung or lobe;
- pneumothorax;
- pleural effusion;
- pleural thickening.

Breath sounds may be bronchial over the upper border of a pleural effusion, or over pulmonary collapse when the surrounding lung is collapsed around open large airways.

Added sounds

The commonest added sounds are crackles and wheezes. This terminology has replaced the older terminology of crepitations or râles and rhonchi respectively, being much less confusing.

Examination Crackles are discontinuous sounds present on inspiration. They represent abrupt opening of closed small airways.

Wheezes are continuous sounds that are present on inspiration and expiration. They represent oscillations in airflow, produced like a reed instrument, due to airway narrowing, which is usually caused by asthma or bronchitis.

Pleural inflammation may give rise to a creaking sound

known as a pleural rub over the parietal pleura as it moves over the visceral pleura during respiration.

Causes of crackles Small airway closure tends to occur at the bases of the lungs in the recumbent or seated patient due to gravity. It is not uncommon in relatively inert elderly patients and is abolished by deep breathing. Crackles are heard in:

- pulmonary oedema;
- pneumonia;
- bronchitis;
- bronchiectasis;
- fibrosis.

Causes of wheezes A single obstruction such as a foreign body or a carcinoma may give rise to a single inspiratory wheeze — or, if in the larynx, trachea or main bronchus, a loud coarse wheeze or stridor on expiration as well as inspiration.

Common causes of a pleural rub These are:

- infection, which may be limited to the pleura (usually a viral infection);
- infection involving the underlying lung (usually bacterial);
- infarction of the lung due to pulmonary embolism.

Tactile fremitus

Examination Transmission of sounds through the chest wall can be detected by palpating for vibrations as the patient talks. This is called tactile fremitus. Tactile fremitus may be assessed during palpation of the chest, but this is often more useful at the end of the examination to confirm the presence of any abnormality. Ask the patient to repeat a phrase such as 'ninety-nine' as the palm of your hand rests on their chest, and compare the vibrations felt from the right and left side in turn.

Causes The vibrations felt are increased by consolidation (pneumonia) or cavitation of the underlying lung, and reduced by pulmonary collapse or a pleural effusion.

Vocal resonance

Examination To assess vocal resonance repeat the technique described above for tactile fremitus, but listen with a stethoscope.

Causes of abnormalities Vocal resonance is increased in consolidation and, less commonly, in cavitation, and is reduced in pleural effusion.

Whispering pectoriloquy

Examination Ask the patient to whisper '99' or '1, 2, 3, 4' when listening to the chest with a stethoscope.

Causes of increased transmission of sound from the bronchi to the stethoscope (whispering pectoriloquy) are consolidation and rarely at the top of an effusion.

NB: In practice auscultation is best for detecting the fine crackles of pulmonary oedema and expiratory wheeze of airways obstruction (asthma and bronchitis).

Finally, any examination of the chest must include examination of the axillae (for lymph nodes) and breasts (for lumps).

Axillary nodes

Examination Feel for axillary nodes, using the left hand to palpate the right axilla and vice versa. Ask the patient to hold his or her arm loosely at their side; gently feel high into the axilla and then pull the hand down the medial wall, feeling for enlarged nodes which tend to slip out from under your fingertips.

Causes of enlarged nodes

Unilateral Breast carcinoma and infection in the upper limb.

Bilateral Causes of generalized lymphadenopathy — particularly systemic infections (e.g. infectious mononucleosis, cytomegalovirus (CMV), toxoplasmosis), lymphoma and lymphatic leukaemia.

Breasts

Examination For women, first inspect the breasts as the patient holds her arms loosely at her side and then as she presses her hands firmly against her waist to contract the pectoral muscles. Look for lumps, asymmetry of the nipples or dimpling of the skin due to tethering to an underlying carcinoma. Palpate with the flat of the hand the four quadrants of the breast and the axillary tail for lumps.

Causes of abnormalities Any breast lump should be regarded as potentially malignant. Note its consistency, mobility, any tenderness and changes in the overlying skin. The common causes of breast lumps are:
- carcinoma;
- chronic mastitis (with or without cysts);
- fibroadenoma.

Enlargement of the male breast (gynaecomastia) may be physiological, particularly around puberty, or due to drugs (e.g. oestrogens, digoxin, spironolactone) or chronic liver disease (from reduced oestrogen metabolism). Very rarely it is due to carcinoma.

ABDOMINAL EXAMINATION
(Examination box 4, p. 88)

'Is there any pain in the abdomen?'

Technique

When examining the abdomen the position and comfort of both patient and examiner are of paramount importance.

The patient should be as relaxed as possible, lying almost flat — provided they are not limited by pain or orthopnoea — and with the head raised slightly on one pillow (it is very uncomfortable to lie absolutely flat).

The examiner should not need to bend or stoop excessively to perform the examination.

Inspection

First inspect the abdomen during quiet respiration. Look for scars (how recent?), masses, herniae (cough to see if they communicate with intra-abdominal pressure), distension, pulsation, dilated veins and the visible peristalsis of intestinal obstruction.

Causes of abnormal findings Dilated veins suggest inferior vena caval or portal vein obstruction (Fig. 2.11, p. 89). Abdominal distension may be due to any of the five 'f's — fat, fluid, faeces, flatus or fetus.

Examination box 4 **Abdomen**	
Hands	Look for clubbing, bruising (clotting factor defects), spider naevi, palmar erythema and Dupuytren's contracture of chronic liver disease and flap of hepatic encephalopathy
Face	Look for spider naevi and jaundice of chronic liver disease
Conjunctivae and tongue	Look for severe anaemia and jaundice
Neck	Palpate the neck for lymphadenopathy secondary to intra-abdominal carcinoma or lymphoma
Abdomen	Note any tenderness; always ask first. Examine for ascites. Palpate for enlarged organs: liver, spleen, kidneys, colon, and suprapubically for uterus, and ovary. Examine inguinal regions for herniae and nodes. Auscultate for bowel sounds. Perform rectal (and if indicated vaginal) examination. Examine male genitalia for scrotal swellings

Palpation

Before palpating the abdomen (Fig. 2.12, p. 90) ask about pain or tenderness. Throughout the rest of the examination watch the patient's face to ensure that you are not hurting them.

Gently palpate each quadrant of the abdomen, starting away from the site of any pain. Feel for any areas of tenderness or masses, and note if the anterior abdominal wall is rigid due to underlying inflammation.

Tenderness

If there is any tenderness note whether the patient 'guards' the area by tensing surrounding abdominal muscles, and whether tenderness is more marked when pressure is applied or released. Rebound tenderness is tenderness which is more pronounced when deep palpation, often achievable if pressure is increased very slowly, is released suddenly.

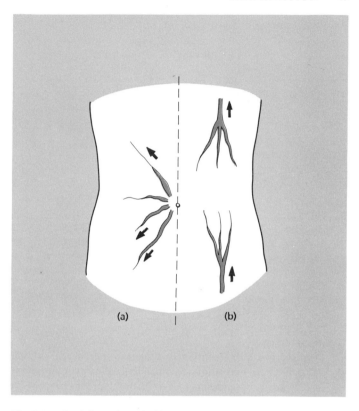

Fig. 2.11 Blood flow through dilated anterior abdominal wall veins.
(a) Direction of flow through dilated abdominal veins in portal vein
occlusion; (b) direction of flow through dilated abdominal veins in
inferior vena caval occlusion. Note that portal vein and inferior vena
caval occlusion can be distinguished by the different directions of flow
below the umbilicus.

Causes Rebound tenderness indicates underlying peritoneal
inflammation, such as from appendicitis or from peritonitis
following rupture of a hollow viscus (e.g. perforated peptic
ulcer) or from pancreatitis.

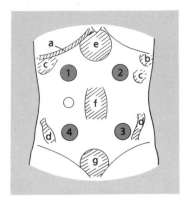

Fig. 2.12 Examination of the abdomen. (i) Gently palpate all quadrants (1–4) for tenderness and masses. (ii) Feel for enlarged: (a) liver, (b) spleen, and (c) kidneys; or masses arising from (d) bowel in the left and right iliac fossae, (e) epigastrium (stomach and pancreas), (f) aorta (aneurysm), (g) pelvis (uterus, bladder and ovaries). (iii) Percuss and auscultate over enlarged organs or masses. (iv) Examine hernial orifices and external genitalia in men. (v) Perform a rectal examination.

Abdominal masses

Examination Palpate any mass to determine its site, size, shape, consistency and mobility, particularly during respiration. Note any tenderness or pulsation, and feel for enlarged lymph nodes in the region of its lymphatic drainage.

Percuss over any masses. The percussion note will be dull over a solid mass. Any overlying bowel will render it resonant.

Causes are shown in Fig. 2.13.

Enlarged organs (liver, spleen, kidneys)

After a general examination of the abdomen for tenderness or masses, examine for enlarged organs.

Liver

Examination The lower border of the liver may be just palpable in thin people on inspiration. The upper border lies between

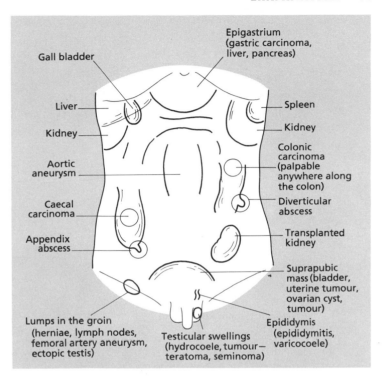

Fig. 2.13 Abdominal masses.

the fourth and fifth rib spaces in the right mid-clavicular line on percussion (see p. 82). The liver enlarges downwards and palpation should start in the right iliac fossa with the fingers lying at right angles to the costal margin (Fig. 2.14, p. 92). Ask the patient to breathe in and out deeply and gradually move the hand upwards during expiration until either the liver or costal margin is felt. The hand should be held still during inspiration, when the liver moves down; if enlarged it will be felt against the fingertips.

Feel the edge of an enlarged liver to determine its texture and regularity and the presence of any tenderness or pulsation.

2

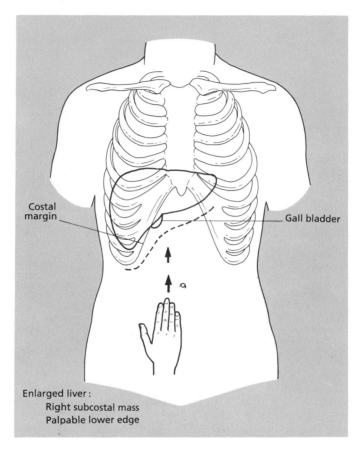

Fig. 2.14 Technique for examining the liver. In an enlarged liver, the palpable lower edge moves with respiration and is dull to percussion. Note that Riedel's lobe and right liver lobe enlargement can be confused with: enlarged right kidney; carcinoma of the hepatic flexure of the colon; and, rarely, enlarged, obstructed and fluid-filled gall bladder.

Determine the position of the lower edge and the level of the upper border by percussion to confirm that the liver is truly enlarged and not just displaced down by over-expansion of the chest.

The scratch test is a useful screening test for liver enlargement. Place the stethoscope in the xiphisternal notch (which is 'always' over liver, normal or abnormal) and find the limits of transmission (through the liver) of a gentle scratch on the skin up and down the right mid-clavicular line in the abdomen.

Common causes of hepatomegaly are:
- cardiac failure;
- secondary carcinomatous deposits;
- cirrhosis.

Other causes include:
- infection — viral (hepatitis, glandular fever), bacterial (liver abscess) or parasitic (amoebic abscess, hydatid cysts);
- reticuloendothelial disorders (leukaemia, myelofibrosis, lymphoma);
- amyloidosis;
- sarcoidosis;
- storage disease (glycogen, lipid);
- primary hepatoma;
- haemochromatosis (increased iron absorption leading to iron deposition in liver and other organs);
- primary biliary cirrhosis;
- Wilson's disease (increased copper deposition).

Riedel's lobe is a normal anatomical variant with enlargement of the right lateral part of the right lobe of the liver.

NB: In cardiac failure the liver is smooth and tender and if tricuspid regurgitation is present it is also pulsatile.

An enlarged liver due to secondary carcinomatous deposits is hard and irregular and usually not tender, while that due to cirrhosis (usually caused by alcohol) is smooth or nodular, hard and not tender.

Spleen

Examination The spleen normally lies under and along the left ninth, tenth and eleventh ribs, and needs to increase two to three times in size before it becomes palpable under the anterior costal margin.

The spleen usually enlarges downwards and diagonally across the abdomen. Palpation should therefore start in the right iliac fossa, into which the spleen may rarely extend (Fig. 2.15).

Gently palpate across the abdomen with the right hand from the right iliac fossa to the left hypochondrium (i.e. the left subcostal region). As the patient breathes in deeply the spleen moves diagonally downwards. The left hand may be placed under the tenth and eleventh ribs posteriorly and pulled to tilt the spleen forward during palpation, and the patient may be asked to roll onto their right side to allow the spleen to fall forwards.

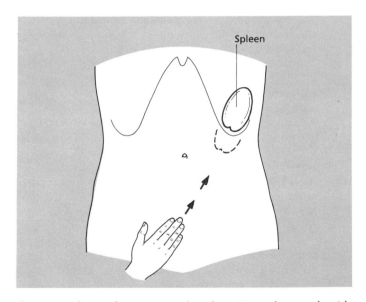

Fig. 2.15 Technique for examining the spleen. Moves downwards with respiration, is dull to percussion and has a palpable notch. The examiner is unable to get a hand between it and the rib cage. It must be differentiated from a left kidney.

If a mass is felt, confirm that it is the spleen by feeling for a notch, establishing that it is not possible to get between it and the rib cage, and demonstrating that the mass is dull to percussion.

Causes of splenomegaly Common causes of massive splenomegaly are:

- chronic myeloid leukaemia;
- myelofibrosis;
- malaria and kala-azar (visceral leishmaniasis).

Common causes of moderate splenomegaly are:

- reticuloendothelial disease;
- cirrhosis with portal hypertension.

Common causes of mild splenomegaly are infections including:

- glandular fever;
- hepatitis;
- brucellosis;
- infective endocarditis.

Rare causes of splenomegaly include amyloidosis, sarcoidosis, storage diseases, connective tissue diseases and splenic abscess.

Kidneys

Examination The left kidney, which lies retroperitoneally on the posterior abdominal wall beneath the diaphragm, is not normally palpable. The lower pole of the right kidney, which lies beneath the liver and is therefore lower than the left, may be felt in thin people (Fig. 2.16, p. 96).

The kidneys should be palpated bimanually with one hand in the loin and the other anteriorly — renal swellings can be felt by pressing the two hands together (ballottement of the kidney). They move slightly downward on inspiration and are resonant to percussion because of overlying bowel gas.

Causes of unilateral renal enlargement

- Carcinoma;
- hydronephrosis;
- cysts;
- compensatory hypertrophy of a single kidney.

2

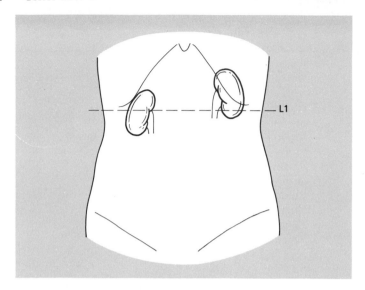

Fig. 2.16 Technique for examining the kidneys. A right or left loin mass moves downwards with respiration, is bimanually palpable and is resonant to percussion. A large right kidney must be differentiated from Riedel's lobe of liver and colonic carcinoma of the hepatic flexure. A large left kidney must be differentiated from a large spleen and colonic carcinoma of the splenic flexure. L1 = level of first lumbar vertebra.

Causes of bilateral renal enlargement
- Polycystic kidneys;
- bilateral hydronephrosis.

Notes Colonic masses due to carcinoma or inflammation usually present as discrete swellings, which may be mobile. Faeces may be indented and tend to disappear between examinations and after enemas.

Masses in the right subcostal region may be from liver (including Riedel's lobe), kidney or the hepatic flexure of the colon.

Masses in the left subcostal region may be from kidney, spleen or splenic flexure of the colon. It may be impossible to distinguish these on clinical grounds alone and without ultrasound. It is better to be uncertain than wrong.

Masses in the groin

Swellings in the groins are usually herniae or lymph nodes.

Understanding inguinal herniae requires a knowledge of the anatomy of the inguinal canal (which contains the spermatic cord in men and the round ligament in women) and the femoral canal (which contains a lymph node and a plug of fat (Fig. 2.17).

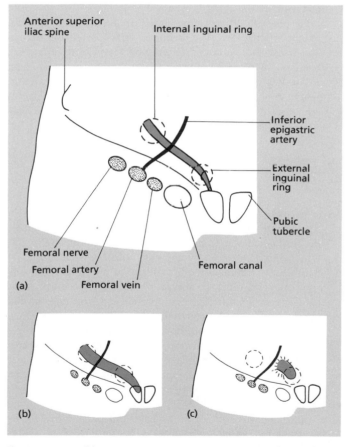

Fig. 2.17 Inguinal herniae. (a) Anatomy; (b) indirect inguinal hernia; (c) direct inguinal hernia.

The neck of an inguinal hernia is above and medial to the pubic tubercle (a distinct, palpable prominence at the lateral border of the pubic crest). If the hernia is indirect it passes along the inguinal canal towards, and sometimes into, the scrotum. If it is direct it pushes the anterior abdominal wall forward above the inguinal ligament.

The neck of a femoral hernia passes through the femoral canal, below and lateral to the pubic tubercle. Strangulation is common as the canal is narrow.

Herniae are either reducible or irreducible, and strangulated or not strangulated. If a hernia is strangulated the hernial sac constricts the contained bowel and restricts its blood supply, resulting in gangrene of the bowel if it is not promptly released.

If a swelling in the groin is elliptical and feels like an inguinal lymph node, look for other nodes along both inguinal ligaments and elsewhere (e.g. in the neck and axillae). Also check for sources of infection in the drainage area of the gland (i.e. in that leg), including between the toes.

Other causes of swelling in the groin are lipoma, aneurysm (femoral artery or saphenous vein) and testicular disease (ectopic testis, hydrocoele of the cord).

Pelvic masses

Bladder enlargement is felt in the mid-line suprapubically, is dull to percussion, and disappears after complete emptying, which can be ensured by catheterization. Distension is usually painful and accompanied by a desire to micturate. These symptoms may, however, be absent, particularly if the urinary retention is long-standing or neuropathic in origin (e.g. in diabetic autonomic neuropathy).

In women, suprapubic pelvic swellings may also arise from the ovaries (cysts, carcinoma) or uterus (fibroids, pregnancy).

The aorta may be palpable in thin people. In the elderly an easily palpable aortic mass may indicate an aortic aneurysm.

Rectal examination (Fig. 2.18)

Rectal examination forms an essential part of the abdominal examination and should always be performed if abdominal pathology is suspected.

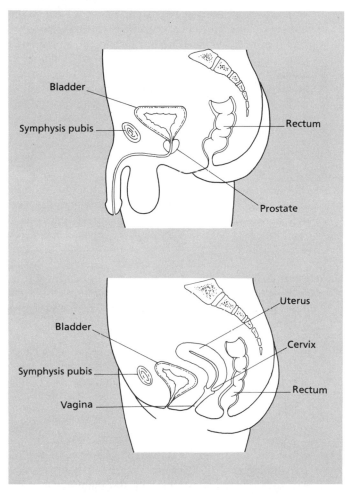

Fig. 2.18 Sagittal sections of the male and female pelvis.

Technique Explain the procedure and reassure the patient, who should lie in the left lateral position with knees bent upwards towards the chest.

Inspect the perianal region for external haemorrhoids or

skin tags (indicating previously thrombosed haemorrhoids). Asking the patient to bear down may further expose haemorrhoids or reveal perianal fissures. Insert the gloved and lubricated index finger gently through the anal sphincter. Feel anteriorly for the prostate gland in men and for the cervix in women. Circle the finger around the rectum to feel for rectal or pelvic masses. On removing the finger note the presence and colour of any faecal material, blood or mucus.

You will be shown how to perform rectal examination during the first clinical phase — if not, ask one of your tutors to help you.

Vaginal examination

Vaginal examination is useful to determine the presence of pelvic masses, particularly uterine or ovarian, but should only be performed supervised by a trained expert. A chaperone should always be present.

Scrotal examination

The scrotum should be examined for the presence of swellings.
Causes of scrotal swelling Scrotal swelling may be testicular or scrotal in origin.
Testicular causes
  • Orchitis (tender swelling, which may be associated with epididymitis and/or urethritis);
  • torsion (abruptly and extremely tender swelling — requires urgent surgical treatment);
  • carcinoma (usually painless and hard).
Scrotal causes
  • Hydrocoele; fluid in tunica vaginalis results in swelling which is translucent if a light is shone from behind (i.e. transillumination) — a feature of clear fluids in general;
  • inguinal hernia (descends from the inguinal canal in front of the spermatic cord).

Ascites (pp. 327 and 340)

Ascites is free fluid in the peritoneal cavity. Usually 2−3 litres need to be present before it is clinically detectable.

Examination When lying supine, ascitic fluid collects in the flanks and can be demonstrated by the presence of 'shifting dullness' or a 'fluid thrill'. First percuss over the flank for dullness — if the flank is resonant, fluid is not present in clinically detectable quantities.

If the flank is dull to percussion, demonstrate the presence of free fluid by asking the patient to roll onto the other side, towards which the fluid will then drain. The site that was originally percussed will then become resonant. This is called shifting dullness (Fig. 2.19).

To demonstrate a fluid thrill (Fig. 2.20, p. 102) ask the patient or a colleague to place the edge of their hand firmly along the mid-line of the abdomen to prevent transmission of impulses through fat or skin. If fluid is present within the peritoneal cavity a firm tap or flick of the finger on one side of the abdomen is transmitted across the peritoneal cavity and felt by the examiner's palm resting on the other flank.

Abdominal auscultation

Listen for the presence of bowel sounds by placing the stethoscope just above and below the umbilicus.

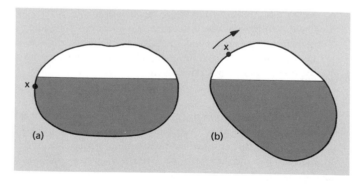

Fig. 2.19 Demonstrating shifting dullness. Cross-section through fluid-filled abdomen. 'X' is dull to percussion on lying flat (a) but resonant on turning the patient (b).

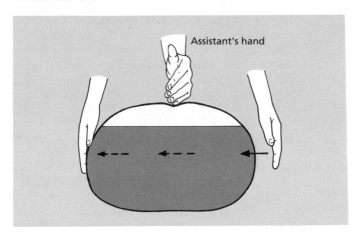

Fig. 2.20 Eliciting a fluid thrill. Cross-section through a fluid-filled abdomen.

Causes of abnormal bowel sounds Bowel sounds are completely absent in:
- peritonitis, which is usually obvious clinically from the associated board-like abdominal rigidity and marked tenderness;
- paralytic ileus, which is an absence of bowel peristalsis and usually follows surgery, lasting 24–48 hours depending upon the amount of intestinal manipulation during the operation. Less commonly it occurs with electrolyte disturbances (e.g. hypokalaemia — low potassium).

In bowel obstruction, the bowel sounds become high-pitched and tinkling.

Causes of bruits Bruits in the abdomen indicate arterial disease and may be heard with the stethoscope over stenosed renal arteries, over atheromatous narrowing of the coeliac or femoral arteries and over abdominal aortic aneurysms.

EXAMINATION OF THE NERVOUS SYSTEM
(Examination box 5, p. 103) (Figs 2.21, 2.22, 2.23)

Because of the complexity of the nervous system a thorough and systematic, yet rapid, examining technique must be adopted.

Examination box 5
Central nervous system

History	A carefully taken history is critical to assess mental state, anxiety, depression or mental impairment. Question in more detail if indicated
Higher cerebral function	Assess using questions and answers (e.g. address, telephone number, Prime Minister's name) and the Babcock sentence
Cranial nerves	Test for smell (I). Examine the eyes (II, III, IV, VI, VIII). Test facial sensation (V). Test facial muscles (VII). Examine the mouth (V). Examine the tongue (XII) and palate (IX, X). Test the neck muscles and trapezius (XI). Test hearing (VIII)
Upper limbs	Look for obvious wasting, paralysis and fasciculation. Check posture by observing outstretched hands for drifting in upper motor neurone lesions. Test: <ul><li>tone</li><li>power (shoulder flexion and extension, elbow flexion and extension, wrist flexion and extension, and small hand muscles)</li><li>reflexes (biceps, triceps and supinator)</li><li>sensation</li><li>coordination (finger–nose test)</li><li>for dysdiadochokinesia</li></ul>
Lower limbs	Look for wasting, paralysis and fasciculation. Test: <ul><li>tone</li><li>power (hip flexion and extension, knee flexion and extension, and ankle flexion and extension)</li><li>reflexes (knee jerk, ankle jerk, plantar responses)</li><li>sensation</li><li>coordination (heel–shin test)</li></ul>
Posture	Observe standing posture with eyes open and closed (Romberg's test). Look for ataxia when walking normally and heel to toe

2

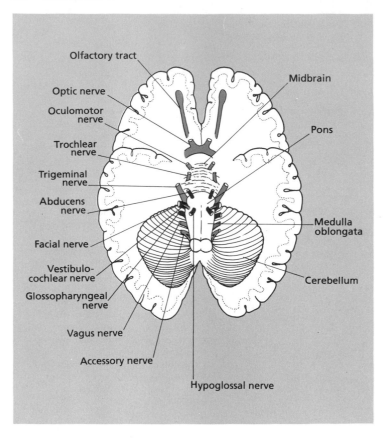

Fig. 2.21 Cranial nerves on inferior surface of brain.

This can be achieved only by repeated practice on patients with both normal and abnormal nervous systems, until the procedure becomes second nature.

Although part of a continuum, the examination can be considered in three sections:
- higher cerebral function;
- cranial nerves;
- limbs.

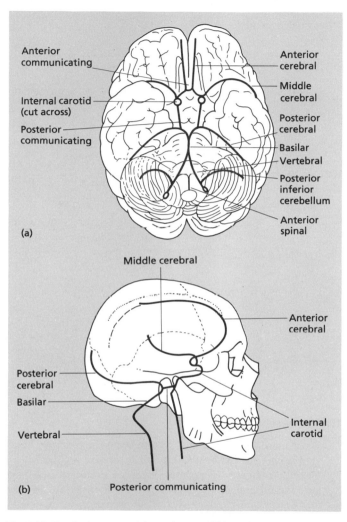

Fig. 2.22 Cerebral arteries. (a) Basal view; (b) lateral view.

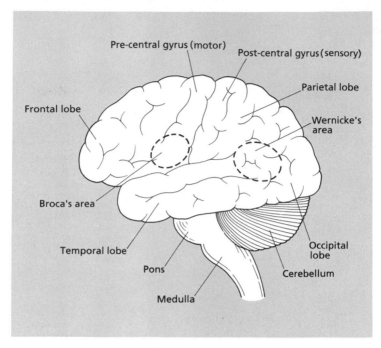

Fig. 2.23 Lateral aspect of the cerebral hemispheres.

Higher cerebral function

Examination of the nervous system begins on meeting the patient
and taking the history. Their ability to give a coherent history
usually indicates a normal level of consciousness, speech,
orientation and intellectual function. If there are any doubts,
higher cerebral function should be examined in more detail.

Conscious level

Examination The level of consciousness ranges from fully alert
to totally unresponsive to stimuli.

If the level of consciousness is depressed it is important to define accurately how responsive the patient is. Determine whether the patient is rousable by talking loudly or by shaking him/her. If not, look for any response, either appropriate or inappropriate, to unpleasant or painful stimuli by pinching the skin, pressing and rubbing the sternum with a knuckle, or pressing firmly over the supraorbital nerve in its notch medially in the eyebrow. Feel for the notch by palpating along the supraorbital ridge. All of these can give considerable pain without damaging tissue.

Glasgow Coma Scale

Changes in the patient's conscious level may be charted using the Glasgow Coma Scale:

Eye opening
1 None.
2 To pain.
3 To speech.
4 Spontaneous.

Best verbal response
1 None.
2 Incomprehensible.
3 Inappropriate.
4 Confused.
5 Orientated.

Best motor response
1 None.
2 Extending.
3 Flexing.
4 Localizing.
5 Obeying.

Patients are scored for each of the three categories. The sum of the three scores gives a measure of their overall conscious level, the range being from 3 (completely unresponsive) to 14 (fully conscious).

Causes of abnormal level of consciousness Commonly loss of consciousness follows head injuries, intracerebral bleeding and thrombosis (strokes) and cerebral infection (meningitis and encephalitis). Varying degrees also occur in all system failures — respiratory and cardiac from hypoxia, renal and liver failure from circulating tissue metabolites. Diabetes (hypoglycaemia, ketoacidosis or hyperosmolar), epilepsy and drug overdose must always be considered.

Remember

Accident (head injury or cerebrovascular)

Epilepsy

Insulin (excess or deficiency) and Infection

Overdose

Uraemia (and other system failures)

Intellectual function

Examination If the patient's speech or behaviour suggests impairment of cognitive function:

• ask the patient their name, the date and where they are, in order to assess orientation;

• ask the patient to tell you the name of the Prime Minister and to recount recent events in the news and distant events relating to their childhood, in order to assess memory.

Loss of memory for recent more than distant events is a feature of dementia.

Concentration and mental function

Examination Interpretation of concentration and mental function must be related to the patient's background and expected ability. Various tests are available and include the following:

• serial sevens — ask the patient to subtract sevens serially from 100;

• repetition of numbers forwards and backwards — most people can remember five or more forwards and four or more backwards;

• repetition of complex sentences such as the Babcock sentence — 'The one thing a nation requires to be rich and famous is a large secure supply of wood';

• interpretation of proverbs such as 'every cloud has a silver lining', 'people who live in glass houses shouldn't throw stones'.

Causes of reduced concentration and mental function The commonest causes in the elderly are Alzheimer's disease and multi-infarct dementia. Other causes are: subdural haematoma, malignancy (primary cerebral tumour or secondary), hypothyroidism (myxoedema madness), overmedication (particularly with sedatives), vitamin B_{12} deficiency, multiple sclerosis and AIDS.

Speech

Examination Speech may be affected by impaired articulation (slurred speech or dysarthria) or impaired comprehension or expression (receptive or expressive dysphasia or aphasia). The comprehension and expression of speech are controlled by the dominant cerebral hemisphere, which is the left hemisphere in right-handed people and in about 50% of left-handed people.

Causes of dysarthria Dysarthria results from neuromuscular lesions involving the oropharynx or larynx and does not imply any defect of intellectual function.

Causes of dysphasia and aphasia Impaired comprehension of speech is receptive dysphasia and results from lesions of the temporoparietal lobes (Wernicke's area). It can be tested for by asking the patient to perform simple commands.

Inability to formulate words or sentences despite being able to comprehend speech and knowing what to say is expressive dysphasia. It results from lesions in the lower pre-central gyrus of the frontal lobes (Broca's area).

Nominal dysphasia is a particular form of expressive dysphasia characterized by an inability to name objects. It can be tested by showing the patient objects and asking him or her to name them. For example, hold up a pen and ask 'What is this?' If the patient is unable to answer, prompt him or her by saying 'Is it a watch? book? pen?' The patient will then identify the correct answer.

Cranial nerves (Examination box 6, p. 110; Fig. 2.21)

The cranial nerves should be examined individually, remembering their anatomy and function. A suggested routine for their examination is given in Examination box 6 on p. 110.

Examination box 6
Suggested routine for examining the cranial nerves

Sense	What to test	Cranial nerve involved
Smell	Ask about sense of smell	I
Eyes	Visual acuity and fields	II
	Pupil reflexes to light and accommodation	II, III
	Fundoscopy	II
	External ocular movements	III, IV, VI
	(observing for nystagmus)	VIII
Facial sensation	Test three divisions with cottonwool and pin	V
	Corneal reflexes	V (VII)
Facial muscles	'Wrinkle your forehead'	VII
	'Screw up your eyes'	
	'Show me your teeth'	
Mouth	'Clench your teeth' (feeling masseters)	V
	'Open your mouth and move your jaw from side to side' (pterygoids)	
	Say 'Ah'	X (IX)
Tongue	Observe in mouth, and protruded	XII
Neck	'Shrug your shoulders'	XI
	'Put your chin on your right (left) shoulder'	
Ears	Test hearing, perform Rinné and Weber tests	VIII
	Examine external canal and tympanic membrane	

Cranial nerve I — the olfactory nerve

Anatomy See Anatomy box 1, p. 111.

Examination Ask the patient whether they have noticed any recent change in sense of smell. If so, test their ability to differentiate smells, using 'smell bottles', separately for each nostril. Use vanilla essence and cloves and avoid strong agents which give rise to non-olfactory stimuli (e.g. ammonia).

Causes of lesions Lesions of the olfactory nerve are rare. The commonest cause of the loss of the sense of smell is local

Anatomy box 1
Olfactory nerve

Fibres arise from the olfactory receptors in the upper nasal cavity
In order, they then:
• pass through the cribriform plate of the ethmoid bone to the
olfactory bulb lying under the frontal lobe
• radiate via the olfactory tract to the temporal cortex

Anatomy box 2
Optic nerve

The optic nerve in order:
• leaves the orbit through the optic foramen accompanied by the
ophthalmic artery
• joins the contralateral optic nerve at the optic chiasma where fibres
from the temporal visual fields cross
• continues as the optic tract to the lateral geniculate body
• relays via the optic radiation to the optic cortex (for visual
perception), and to the oculomotor (third cranial) nerve nucleus and
medial longitudinal bundle (for pupil reflexes and control of eye
movements)

disease in the nasal passages (e.g. colds and rhinitis) and the
commonest neurological lesion is head trauma.

Cranial nerve II – the optic nerve

Anatomy See Anatomy box 2 (above).

Examination Examination of the optic nerve should start with
an assessment of visual acuity. This may be tested by asking
the patient to distinguish distant objects or read print, and
can be formally assessed, for each eye, using Snellen type (for
distant vision) and Jaegar (for near vision). Refractive errors
should be corrected by allowing the patient to wear their
spectacles.

Visual fields (Fig. 2.24)

Assess the patient's visual fields by comparing them with your
own. Sit the patient at arm's length directly in front of you and

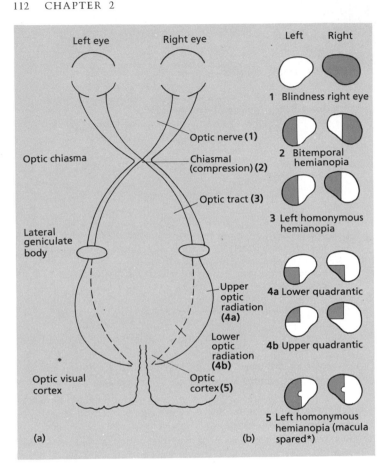

Fig. 2.24 Lesions of the optic nerve and tract and effects on visual fields. (a) Anatomical lesion; (b) visual field defect. ˙ The macula has extensive cortical representation and may be spared by lesions of the visual cortex.

ask them to cover their right eye as you cover your left. Then ask them to look directly into your pupil as you bring an object such as a the head of a hat pin from the periphery of each of the four quadrants of the visual field (right and left, upper and lower) towards the centre and to say when they first see the pin. Neither you nor the patient should be able to see the pin when you start.

Compare the extent of the patient's visual fields with your own. Defects within the field of vision ('scotoma') can be tested by passing a large pinhead across the centre of the visual field and asking when it disappears and reappears. In each central field there is a normal scotoma (blind spot), medial to the point at which the patient is looking (point of fixation), which corresponds to the optic disc, in which there are no visual receptors. It increases in size if the optic disc is swollen (papilloedema).

Pupillary reflexes

Shining a light on the retina constricts the pupil on the same side (the direct-light pupil reflex) and the pupil on the opposite side (the consensual-light pupil reflex). The reflex arc involves the optic nerve, the optic tract, the lateral geniculate nuclei, the parasympathetic component of the oculomotor nerve (Edinger −Westphal nucleus), and the ciliary nerves via the ciliary ganglion. When testing the light reflex the torch should be flashed twice at each eye (once for the direct and once for the consensual reflex), preferably from the side to avoid eliciting an accommodation reflex.

Focusing on a near object results in the accommodation reflex, which comprises contraction of the ciliary muscles, convergence of the eyes and constriction of the pupil. Ask the patient to look at a distant object, and then to focus on a near object, such as your finger, held 6−12 inches away from their face. The reflex arc involves the occipital cortex and the oculomotor nerve nucleus (i.e. it goes through the cerebral cortex).

Optic fundi (Fig. 2.25)

Skill in using the ophthalmoscope to examine the fundi can only be achieved by repeated practice (practice on each other).

Start by turning on the light and check that there is a neat bright circle of light if it is shone on your palm.

The right eye is used for examination of the patient's right fundus, and the left eye for the left fundus. If you normally wear glasses it is easiest to remove them and use the correction

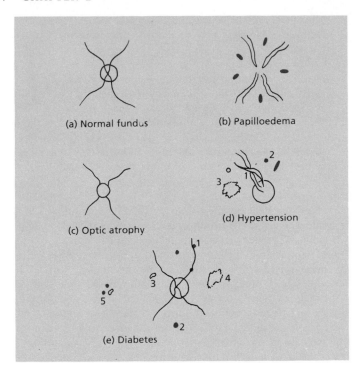

Fig. 2.25 Abnormalities of the optic fundus. (a) Normal fundus.
(b) Papilloedema: swollen disc; dilated tortuous veins; scattered
haemorrhages. (c) Optic atrophy: 'punched-out' disc with marked pallor.
(d) Hypertension: 1, vascular changes — arterial thickening due to
atherosclerosis causes a 'silver wire' appearance and arteriovenous
'nipping'; 2, 'flame' haemorrhages; 3, exudates. (e) Diabetes:
1, microaneurysms; 2, 'dot and blot' haemorrhages; 3, hard exudates
(protein leaking into retina); 4, soft exudates (retinal ischaemia/
infarction); 5, 'maculopathy' — haemorrhages and exudates in macula
region: cause severe visual loss.

lens in the ophthalmoscope to correct for your own refractive
error. Sit the patient in a darkened room and ask them to focus
on a fixed point on the ceiling. Then look through the ophthal-

moscope from a distance at the patient's eye, keeping the machine close to your eye and ensuring that it moves with movements of your head.

Your head and the ophthalmoscope must be considered as one unit – practise by looking around the room – otherwise it is impossible to fix on the retina. Set the ophthalmoscope at +15 or +20 so that the iris and lens are in focus and there is only a blurred red reflex of light reflected from the retina. Cataracts appear as opacities in the red reflex. Then, gradually turn the ophthalmoscope lens towards zero so that the vitreous and then the retina come into focus. Once one of the retinal vessels is seen, focus sharply on it by further adjusting the lenses, and follow it inwards towards the optic disc. Examine the disc and retina in detail and then ask the patient to look directly at the light to examine the macula.

Causes of visual field defects depend upon the site of the lesion (Fig. 2.24, p. 112).

Causes of abnormal pupil responses Absence of the light reflex may result from lesions anywhere in the reflex arc or be a result of drugs (e.g. opiates). Loss of the direct-light reflex with preservation of the consensual reflex implies that the lesion lies on the afferent or sensory side of the reflex arc. Such lesions may involve the eye itself.

Loss of the light reflex with retention of the accommodation reflex (e.g. Argyll Robertson pupils of tertiary syphilis, which is now very rare) occurs with lesions of the brain stem or ciliary ganglion.

Loss of the accommodation reflex with preservation of the light reflex implies a lesion of the occipital cortex.

Causes of lesions of the sympathetic nerves (see Anatomy box 3, p. 116) Paralysis of the sympathetic nerves at any site in the cervical chain may be due to:
- vascular lesions;
- compression;
- demyelination.

This results in Horner's syndrome, which is characterized by
- enophthalmos (the eyeball is indrawn);
- meiosis (small pupil);
- ptosis (drooping of the upper lid);

Anatomy box 3
Sympathetic nerves to the eye

Sympathetic nerves supplying the eye arise in the hypothalamus

Preganglionic fibres
Pass through the pons and medulla and exit with the anterior nerve
roots of C8 and T1 to the superior cervical ganglion

Postganglionic fibres
Pass in the carotid sheath with the internal carotid artery through the
cavernous sinus to join the ophthalmic branch of the trigeminal nerve;
supply smooth muscle fibres of levator palpebrae superioris and dilator
pupillae, and cause facial vasodilatation and sweating

- anhydrosis (decreased sweating over the affected side of the face);
- that is, everything gets smaller or contracts.

Common abnormalities of the optic fundus are shown in Fig. 2.25, p. 114.

Causes of papilloedema

- Raised intracranial pressure (cerebral tumour, cerebral abscess, meningitis, rarely 'benign intracranial hypertension' in young women);
- malignant hypertension;
- retinal vein obstruction (central retinal vein thrombosis, cavernous sinus thrombosis);
- optic neuritis (inflammation of the optic nerve, most commonly due to multiple sclerosis);
- rarely, metabolic causes (carbon dioxide (CO_2) retention in respiratory failure, hypoparathyroidism).

Causes of optic atrophy

- Prolonged papilloedema from any cause;
- optic neuritis;
- interference with the blood supply to the optic nerve (retinal artery occlusion);
- compression of the optic nerve – intraocular (glaucoma) or extraocular (e.g. tumour, aneurysm, trauma);
- rarely methanol abuse, vitamin B_{12} deficiency, hereditary ataxias.

Cranial nerves III (oculomotor nerve), IV (trochlear nerve) and VI (abducent nerve)

Cranial nerves III, IV and VI are usually examined together.

Anatomy (see Anatomy box 4, below) Muscles involved in eye movement are shown in Fig. 2.26 on p. 118.

Anatomy box 4
Oculomotor, trochlear and abducent nerves

Oculomotor nerve
Nucleus lies in the mid-brain
Fibres pass forward across the posterior fossa and through the cavernous
    sinus to the orbit
Supplies all extraocular muscles except superior oblique, lateral rectus,
    levator palpebrae superioris and sphincter pupillae

Trochlear nerve
Nucleus lies just anterior to the oculomotor nerve nucleus in the
    mid-brain
Fibres pass backwards and inwards, crossing over, and leaving the
    posterior aspect of the mid-brain they pass through the cavernous
    sinus to the orbit
Supplies the superior oblique, which depresses the eye, particularly
    when it is turned medially

Abducent nerve
Nucleus lies in the pons
Passes forward through the cerebellopontine angle and cavernous sinus
    to the orbit
Supplies the lateral rectus, which moves the eye outwards

Examination To test eye movements ask the patient to fix their gaze on an object, such as the examiner's finger or the head of a hat pin. Move the object to both sides and then, with the eye in central, medial and lateral positions, move it upwards and downwards.

Test both eyes together and ask the patient to say if they see double and to describe the separation. If double vision occurs, the image furthest from the mid-line arises from the affected eye. This can be identified by asking the patient to cover each eye in turn and say which image disappears.

When testing eye movements look for nystagmus, which is

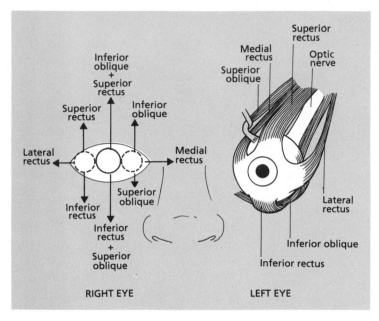

Fig. 2.26 Eye movements.

a repetitive oscillation of the eye. It is usually composed of a quick 'jerky' phase in one direction followed by a slower return in the opposite direction. The direction of the quick phase is arbitrarily taken as the 'direction' of the nystagmus. Occasionally nystagmus may be 'pendular', when the speed of both phases of oscillation is equal.

As the levator palpebrae superioris is supplied by the superior ramus of the oculomotor nerve, look for ptosis (drooping of the upper eyelid).

A lesion of the oculomotor nerve causes the eye to move 'down and out'. In addition the pupil is dilated and ptosis is present.

Causes of diplopia If the images are separated laterally and are parallel the cause is almost invariably a lateral rectus (sixth nerve) palsy; if the separation between the images is angulated the cause is probably a superior oblique palsy (fourth nerve).

Palsies of the extraocular muscles cause double vision (diplopia) which is maximal on moving the eye in the direction in which it is normally moved by the affected muscle.

Causes of nystagmus The causes of 'jerky' nystagmus are:

- lesions of the vestibular nerve or its connections when it is maximal on looking away from the side of a destructive lesion;
- cerebellar lesion when it is greater on looking towards the side of a destructive lesion.

The causes of 'pendular' nystagmus are usually ocular conditions that impair visual fixation (e.g. very short sight).

Causes of ptosis

- Oculomotor nerve lesions (when it is usually complete);
- sympathetic nerve lesions as part of a Horner's syndrome (when it is usually partial);
- primary muscle diseases (e.g. myasthenia gravis, dystrophia myotonica).

Cranial nerve V – the trigeminal nerve

The trigeminal nerve is composed of a motor component, which supplies the muscles of mastication (masseters, temporalis and pterygoids), and a sensory component, which supplies the face and sinuses.

Anatomy See Anatomy box 5, p. 120.

Examination (motor component) Feel the bulk of the masseters and temporal muscles and test the muscles by asking the patient:

- to clench their jaw (masseters and temporals);
- to move the jaw from side to side and to keep it open against pressure (pterygoids).

Weakness causes deviation to the same side.

To elicit the jaw jerk ask the patient to let their mouth hang open while you hold their chin between your thumb and forefinger. Tapping your thumb with a tendon hammer results in an upward jerking of the chin.

Examination (sensory component) Test sensation to light touch with a wisp of cotton wool. Compare the two sides of the face in turn.

The corneal reflex is elicited by touching the side of the cornea (not the sclera) with a wisp of cotton wool, causing

Anatomy box 5
Trigeminal nerve

Motor component
Nucleus lies in the mid-pons
Fibres pass with the sensory fibres from the lateral border of the pons,
    through the cerebellopontine angle into the petrous temporal bone,
    where they pass below the sensory Gasserian ganglion, leaving the
    skull through the foramen ovale
Supplies the masseters, pterygoids and temporal muscles

Sensory component
Three branches which meet in the Gasserian ganglion
I The ophthalmic (first) division supplies the forehead, anterior half of
    the scalp, the root of the nose, the cornea and the conjunctiva and
    enters the skull through the cavernous sinus

II The maxillary (second) division supplies the nose, cheek, upper teeth
    and gums, and the hard and soft palates and enters the skull through
    the foramen rotundum

III The mandibular (third) division enters the skull through the foramen
    ovale. It supplies the skin of the jaw, the mucosa of the cheek, the
    jaw, the floor of the mouth and the anterior two-thirds of the tongue
        Fibres terminate in an area extending from the pons, through
    the medulla, to the third cervical segment

both eyes to blink. It depends upon intact corneal sensation
and an intact facial nerve, which supplies orbicularis oculi. If
the facial nerve is paralysed on one side, the contralateral eye
will still blink.

Causes of jaw muscle weakness The muscles on each side
    receive fibres from both motor nuclei. Unilateral weakness
    therefore indicates a lower motor neurone lesion (i.e. damage
    to the unilateral fifth nerve or its nucleus).

Causes of an abnormal jaw jerk The jaw jerk is exaggerated in
    bilateral upper motor neurone lesions.

Cranial nerve VII — the facial nerve

Anatomy See Anatomy box 6, p. 121.

Examination Test facial muscles by asking the patient to:

Anatomy box 6
Facial nerve

Arises in the pons

Passes around the abducens (sixth cranial) nerve nucleus and exits at the cerebellopontine angle

It then enters the facial canal through the internal auditory meatus with the vestibulocochlear (eighth cranial) nerve and enlarges in the canal to form the geniculate ganglion

The geniculate ganglion receives sensory fibres from the external ear and taste fibres from the lingual branch of the trigeminal nerve via the chorda tympani

From the geniculate ganglion, fibres leave as:
- the nerve to stapedius
- the greater petrosal nerve to the lacrimal glands
- the lesser petrosal nerve to the submandibular and sublingual glands

Remaining fibres leave the facial canal to pass around the angle of the jaw through the parotid gland to supply all the facial muscles except levator palpebrae superioris

2

- wrinkle their forehead (frontalis);
- screw up the eyes (orbicularis oculi);
- blow out the cheeks (buccinator);
- whistle (orbicularis oris);
- show their gums or teeth (levator anguli oris and risorius).

Causes of lesions Because of the anatomical relationships of the facial nerve, lesions can be accurately located.

Fibres to the upper facial muscles are represented on both sides of the cerebral cortex and forehead movements are therefore retained in upper motor neurone lesions ('upper spares upper' in strokes).

Lower motor neurone lesions (Bell's palsy) affect both the upper and lower facial muscles.

Lesions in the pons usually give rise to both sixth and seventh nerve palsies because of the close proximity of their nuclei at this site.

Lesions of the geniculate ganglion (e.g herpes zoster infection — Ramsay Hunt syndrome) cause hyperacusis (accentuated sense of hearing) due to involvement of the nerve to stapedius and loss of taste over the anterior two-thirds of the tongue due to involvement of the chorda tympani.

Cranial nerve VIII — the vestibulocochlear nerve

Anatomy See Anatomy box 7 (below).

Anatomy box 7
Vestibulocochlear nerve

Two components: cochlear nerve and vestibular nerve
The two components join to enter the skull through the internal
    auditory meatus
The nerve then passes into the brain stem through the cerebellopontine
    angle to divide again into its two components

Cochlear nerve
Arises from the organ of Corti
Ends in dorsal and ventral nuclei in the pons. Here there are connections
    between the two sides of the brain stem
From here fibres relay to the temporal cortex

Vestibular nerve
Arises from the vestibular apparatus (semicircular canals, saccule and
    utricle)
Ends in the upper medulla
From here fibres relay to the cerebellum, third, fourth and sixth nerves
    via the medial longitudinal bundle, and vestibulospinal tract in the
    cord

Examination Hearing can be tested simply by holding a ticking watch, or whispering, close to each ear.

A high-frequency (256 or 512 Hz) tuning fork is used to distinguish conductive from sensorineural deafness as follows:

Rinné's test To perform Rinné's test place the base of a vibrating tuning fork behind the ear on the mastoid process and then rapidly move it so that its prongs are in line with the external auditory meatus. Ask the patient to tell you in which position it is loudest. Normally air conduction is better than bone conduction (Rinné positive). If there is conductive deafness the reverse is true (Rinné negative).

Weber's test To perform Weber's test place a vibrating tuning fork in the middle of the patient's forehead and ask where the sound is heard. It is normally heard in the middle of the forehead or all over (Weber central). If there is nerve deafness it is heard in the unaffected ear. If there is conductive deafness the sound is heard better in the affected ear, which is not 'distracted' by external sounds. Test it yourself by placing a vibrating tuning fork in the middle of your forehead, and then close off one ear with your finger — you have simulated conductive deafness and the sound is transmitted to that ear.

Both conductive and sensorineural deafness may be accompanied by tinnitus (ringing in the ears; see p. 35).

The external ear and tympanic membrane should be examined with an auriscope. Pull the auricle upwards and backwards to straighten the external auditory meatus and inspect it before inserting the speculum. Wax commonly obscures the view and may be removed by syringeing, providing there is no history of middle ear disease.

The normal ear drum (Fig. 2.27, p. 124) is pearl grey in colour with the handle of the malleus running across it and a bright cone of light (known as the light reflex) radiating forward from its lower end.

Damage to the vestibular apparatus or nerve causes vertigo — a sensation of movement, either of self or surroundings, resulting in disturbed balance. The principal physical manifestations are:

• nystagmus, which should be looked for on examination of the ocular movements;

• unsteadiness of gait, with a tendency to stagger towards the side of the lesion.

Causes of hearing abnormalities Deafness may be conductive, due to disease of the middle or external ear (e.g. otitis media, wax), or sensorineural, due to damage affecting the inner ear or auditory nerve.

Causes of ear drum abnormalities Common abnormalities are:

• perforation of the drum;

• otitis media (infection in the middle ear), which causes dullness of the drum and loss of the light reflex at first,

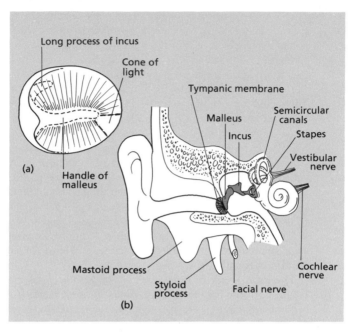

Fig. 2.27 (a) Tympanic membrane as seen through otoscope;
(b) anatomy of the ear.

followed later by reddening and bulging of the drum, and
progressing to perforation if not treated.

Causes of vestibular nerve damage Ototoxic drugs (e.g aminoglycosides such as gentamicin, tobramycin), tumours (acoustic
neuroma or local infiltrating neoplasms), trauma, infection
(meningitis, osteomyelitis of the petrous temporal bone), or
Paget's disease affecting the petrous temporal bone.

Cranial nerves IX (glossopharyngeal nerve) and X (vagus nerve)

Both the glossopharyngeal and vagus nerves are mixed motor
and sensory and serve the oropharynx. For practical purposes IX
is sensory to the pharynx (and a little motor) and X is motor
(and a little sensory). They are examined together.

Anatomy See Anatomy box 8, p. 125.

Anatomy box 8
Glossopharyngeal and vagus nerves

Glossopharyngeal nerve

Arises with the vagus nerve in the nucleus ambiguus in the medulla and leaves the skull with the vagus nerve and the accessory (eleventh) nerve through the jugular foramen

Carries sensory fibres from the nasopharynx, soft palate and posterior two-thirds of the tongue (including taste), and parasympathetic fibres to the parotid gland

Supplies only the stylopharyngeus muscle so its motor function cannot be tested in isolation

Vagus nerve

Arises with the glossopharyngeal nerve in the nucleus ambiguus in the medulla and leaves the skull with the glossopharyngeal nerve and the accessory (eleventh) nerve through the jugular foramen

Passes from the jugular foramen into the neck, chest and abdomen

Carries sensory fibres from part of the external auditory meatus and has extensive afferent and efferent connections with the thoracic and abdominal viscera

Motor fibres supply the soft palate, pharynx and, via the recurrent laryngeal nerve, which loops around the aortic arch on the left, the intrinsic muscles of the larynx

2

Examination The sensory component of the glossopharyngeal nerve and motor component of the vagus nerve can be tested together by eliciting the gag reflex — touching the posterior wall of the pharynx results in its elevation. The procedure is slightly uncomfortable.

The motor component of the vagus can be tested in isolation by asking the patient to say 'Ah' whilst observing for symmetrical upward movement of the soft palate and uvula. If a lesion is present they deviate away from the side of the lesion and there is 'curtain movement' of the posterior pharyngeal wall away from the lesion.

Unilateral paralysis of the laryngeal muscles causes hoarseness of the voice, and can be confirmed by finding paralysis of the vocal cord on laryngoscopy.

Causes of lesions Pharyngeal lesions result from disorders of the bulbar nuclei (see bulbar palsy, p. 127).

Cranial nerve XI — the accessory nerve

The accessory nerve is a motor nerve.

Anatomy See Anatomy box 9 (below).

Anatomy box 9
Accessory nerve

Cranial component originates in the ninth and tenth nerves in the nucleus ambiguus

Spinal component originates from the anterior horn cells of the first to the fourth cervical segments

Spinal component enters the skull through the foramen magnum and joins the cranial part to leave the skull through the jugular foramen. The two components then separate

Spinal component supplies the sternomastoid and trapezius

Cranial component blends with the vagus

Examination To examine the accessory nerve observe and feel the bulk of trapezius as the patient shrugs their shoulders. Then observe and palpate the sternomastoids as the patient puts their chin on their chest. Each side is tested separately by asking the patient to rotate their chin towards each shoulder in turn and feeling the bulk of the muscle on the other side.

Causes of lesions See bulbar palsy, p. 127.

Cranial nerve XII — the hypoglossal nerve

The hypoglossal nerve is the motor nerve to the tongue.

Anatomy See Anatomy box 10 (below).

Anatomy box 10
Hypoglossal nerve

Arises in the medulla

Leaves the skull through the anterior condylar foramen (next to the jugular foramen)

Descends in the neck between the carotid artery and jugular vein to the angle of the jaw, where it passes forward to the tongue

---

Examination First examine the tongue inside the widely open mouth and look for wasting and/or fasciculation (spontaneous muscle contractions). Then ask the patient to stick out their tongue; if there is a lesion of the twelfth nerve or its nucleus the tongue deviates towards the side of the lesion as it is pushed out. (The palate is pulled to the strong side and the tongue pushed to the weak side.)

Causes of lesions See bulbar palsy (below).

Bulbar and pseudobulbar palsy

Involvement of the ninth, tenth and twelfth cranial nerves together causes the syndromes of:

• bulbar palsy if a lesion of lower motor neurones is responsible;

• pseudobulbar palsy if a lesion of upper motor neurones is responsible.

As the nerves have bilateral cortical representation pseudobulbar palsy is only a feature of bilateral lesions — usually of the internal capsule and usually bilateral strokes.

The symptoms of bulbar and pseudobulbar palsy are dysarthria, dysphagia and nasal regurgitation.

Examination Lesions of the cranial nerves IX, X, XII are present (see above). In bulbar palsy (upper motor neurone lesions) the tongue is large, floppy and fasciculating. In pseudobulbar palsy (lower motor neurone lesions) the tongue is small and the jaw jerk exaggerated.

Causes Bulbar palsy can be caused by: multiple small strokes, syringomyelia, motor neurone disease, Guillain–Barré syndrome, poliomyelitis.

Pseudobulbar palsy can be caused by: multiple small strokes, syringobulbia, motor neurone disease.

Limbs (Examination box 7, pp. 128–9)

'Is there any pain in your legs or joints?'

It is convenient to consider neurological examination of the limbs in terms of motor and sensory systems.

Examination box 7
Neurological examination of the limbs

ARMS	Observe for muscle wasting and involuntary movements. Test muscle tone at elbow (cogwheeling at wrist). Test muscle power
Shoulder (C5)	'Hold your arms out in front of you and close your eyes.' Look for drifting due to weakness or loss of position sensation
Elbow	
Flexion, biceps (C5, 6)	'Bend your elbow up; don't let me straighten it'
Extension, triceps (C7)	'Now straighten your elbow and push me away'
Wrist (C7)	'Keep your wrist straight; don't let me bend it'
Fingers (C8, T1)	'Grip my fingers hard' (Give the patient only two fingers to grip — he/she may hurt more!)
Ulnar nerve	'Spread your fingers apart, don't let me squash them together'
Median nerve	'Hold your thumb against your little finger and stop me pulling it away'
Reflexes	Biceps, triceps, supinator
Sensation	Test for light touch and pin-prick sensation at least once on the front and back of the upper and lower arms and on each digit. Test position sensation in a finger and vibration sensation on the styloid process. Test coordination — perform the finger–nose test and look for dysdiadochokinesis
LEGS	Observe for muscle wasting and involuntary movements. Test muscle tone at knee. Test muscle power
Hip	
Flexion, iliopsoas (L1, 2)	'Lift your leg up straight.' Push down on the patient's knee
Knee	'Bend your knee, don't let me straighten it.' Pull on
Flexion, other hamstrings (L5, S1, 2)	the patient's ankle with the hand above his/her knee
Extension, quadriceps (L3, 4)	'Now try and straighten your knee.' Push down on the ankle

Ankle

Plantar flexion, calf (S1)	'Push your foot down against my hand'
Dorsiflexion, ant. tibial (L4, 5)	'Push your foot upwards, don't let me pull it down'
Reflexes	Knee and ankle reflexes and plantar response
Sensation	Test for light touch and pin-prick sensation once on the medial and lateral sides of the thigh and calf, dorsum of foot, tip of the big toe and the lateral border of foot. Test vibration sensation on the medial malleolus and, if absent, on the knee and hip. Test position sensation in the big toes. Test coordination — perform the heel–shin test. Finally, ask the patient to stand. Look for truncal ataxia and Rombergism (i.e. more unsteady with eyes closed indicating loss of position sensation)
GAIT	Watch the patient walk and observe for abnormalities of gait
Hemiplegic gait	The leg on the contralateral side to the cerebral damage is rigid and describes a semicircle with the toe scraping the floor (circumduction). There may also be weakness of the ipsilateral arm. It is almost invariably due to a stroke (cerebral haemorrhage or infarction)
Paraplegic gait	'Scissors' gait due to cord lesions resulting in upper motor neurone lesions in both legs and adduction spasm
Parkinsonian	Stooped, small-stepped, shuffling gait. No arm swing. 'Freezing' in doorways gait
Cerebellar gait	Wide-based, unsteady gait with a tendency to stagger towards the side of unilateral destructive lesions
Sensory ataxia	Stepping, stamping gait. The patient looks at the ground and tends to fall if they close their eyes
Foot drop gait	Loss of dorsiflexion of the foot due to lateral popliteal nerve palsy means that the affected leg has to be lifted high to avoid scraping the toe
Musculoskeletal problems (e.g. osteoarthritis of the hip)	May cause abnormalities of gait

2

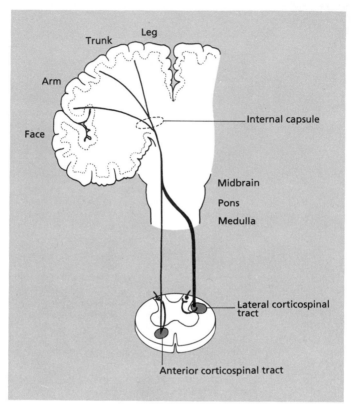

Fig. 2.28 Motor pathways.

Motor system

See Fig. 2.28 above and Anatomy box 11, p. 131.

Examination Motor function assessment of the limbs includes five features:

- muscle wasting (the bulk of muscle groups should be assessed comparing the two sides);
- muscle tone;
- muscle power;

Anatomy box 11
Motor system

Composed of pyramidal and extrapyramidal pathways

Pyramidal fibres (Fig. 2.28, p. 130)
Predominantly involved in precise voluntary movements. They arise
  partly from Betz cells in the pre-frontal convolution, but also from
  more extensive areas of cortex, especially the post-central gyrus
Pyramidal fibres pass through the internal capsule and mid-brain to the
  pons, where most decussate and form the lateral corticospinal tracts.
  A few stay on the same side, forming the anterior corticospinal tracts
The corticospinal tracts continue through the medulla into the spinal
  cord, where they synapse, usually via connecting neurones, with lower
  motor neurones in the anterior horn cells

Extrapyramidal pathways
Involved in learned and habitual movements, such as those associated
  with posture, and the smooth integration of voluntary movements
A complex system of connections between:
  • the corpus striatum (grey matter deep in the cerebral hemispheres)
  • mid-brain structures (basal ganglia)
  • spinal tracts (vestibulospinal and reticulospinal tracts)

2

• coordination and tendon reflexes — compare the two sides;
• involuntary movements.

Muscle wasting
  Examination Look at and feel the muscle bulk, comparing the
  two sides.
  Causes
    • Neuropathic — lower motor neurone lesions (localized due
    to isolated nerve palsies, or part of a generalized neuropathy,
    pp. 38−9);
    • myopathic — primary muscle diseases such as muscular
    dystrophies, metabolic (e.g. diabetes, uraemia, thyroid disease,
    osteomalacia), drugs (e.g. steroids), inflammatory conditions
    (e.g. polymyositis);
    • disuse — either generalized (e.g. following prolonged bed-
    rest) or localized due to joint disease (e.g. around affected

joints in rheumatoid arthritis) or immobilization (e.g. following fractures).

Muscle tone

Examination Assessment of tone is easiest at the elbow and knee and requires the full cooperation and understanding of the patient. Engage the patient in conversation so that they are relaxed and then passively move the joint. Passive movement of a joint normally gives rises to a small amount of resistance due to some reflex contraction of the stretched muscle — this is normal tone.

Roll the outstretched leg and observe how easily the foot rocks on the ankle.

Causes of abnormal tone Increased tone may be due to spasticity or rigidity.

Spasticity is a feature of upper motor neurone (pyramidal) lesions. The increased tone is particularly noticeable on initial movement, but suddenly lessens on continued movement; it is likened to opening a pen-knife — sometimes called 'clasp knife rigidity'.

Rigidity is a feature of extrapyramidal lesions — the increased tone is sustained throughout the range of movement; it is likened to bending a lead pipe — 'lead pipe rigidity'.

In Parkinson's disease the rigidity may be jerky ('cogwheel rigidity') due to superimposed tremor. This is most obvious at the wrist.

Decreased tone (hypotonia, flaccidity) is more difficult to assess. It is a feature of lower motor neurone and cerebellar lesions.

Muscle power

Examination To test muscle power explain the test to the patient ('I am going to test the strength of some of your muscles') and ask them to contract each muscle group against your resistance, comparing the two sides and their strength with your own.

Causes of reduced muscle power These include all of the causes of muscle wasting, together with causes of upper motor neurone lesions (e.g. strokes, demyelination), in which muscle bulk may be preserved.

Coordination

This tests both motor and sensory function.

Examination Muscle weakness and posture in the upper limbs are tested together by asking the patient to hold their arms straight out in front of them with their eyes closed. Upper motor neurone weakness of the proximal limb muscles or loss of postural sense results in a slow drift downwards on the affected side.

Several methods are available for testing coordination.

The finger–nose test To perform the finger–nose test, ask the patient to touch alternately their nose and your finger which you move to different positions within the patient's reach each time.

Test rapid repetitive movements by asking the patient to tap alternately your hand with the front and back of their own hand. Irregularity in the movement is known as dysdiadochokinesis.

The heel–shin test To perform the heel–shin test ask the patient to place their heel on the opposite knee and slide it down the shin to the ankle and back again. Coordination is usually slightly better on the dominant side.

Causes of incoordination

• Abnormal proprioception (sensory ataxia);

• cerebellar lesions (the cerebellum integrates the motor and sensory systems to ensure smooth coordination, but does not design or initiate movement).

Sensory ataxia results from the loss of joint position sense and may be compensated visually. It is therefore exacerbated by closing the eyes. Romberg's test involves standing, preferably with the feet together, first with the eyes open and then with them closed. Rombergism is present if the patient is more unsteady with the eyes closed than open.

Cerebellar ataxia cannot be compensated visually and is often accompanied by tremor (p. 135) and nystagmus (p. 117).

Muscle weakness alone may result in poor coordination.

Tendon reflexes

Examination Details of the principal tendon reflexes are given in Table 2.2, p. 134. Sudden stretching of a muscle — by striking

Table 2.2 Tendon reflexes

Reflex	Muscle involved	Movement	Nerve roots
Biceps	Biceps	Elbow flexion	C 5,6
Supinator	Brachioradialis (previously called supinator longus)	Supination wrist	C 5,6
Triceps	Triceps	Elbow extension	C (6),7,8
Knee	Quadriceps	Knee extension	L 3,4
Ankle	Calf	Plantar flexion	S 1,2

NB: Root value from ankle to triceps = 1,2,3,4,5,6,7 (*aide-mémoire* S1,2 T3,4 C5,6 C7,8).

its tendon — results in reflex contraction of the muscle and movement of the joint. The reflex arc involved is monosynaptic (i.e. afferent sensory fibres from stretch receptors in the muscle synapse directly onto anterior horn cells, activating motor neurones, which return to the stretched muscle and cause contraction) and is modified by higher pathways.

It is essential that the muscle involved is completely relaxed. If it is difficult to elicit a tendon reflex it may be 'reinforced' by asking the patient to concentrate on contracting muscles at a distant site (e.g 'grip your hands together' or 'clench your teeth').

The plantar (Babinski) reflex is elicited by stroking firmly the outer part of the sole of the foot from back to front with a blunt object such as a car key. This reflex is mediated by the first sacral segment of the cord and normally produces plantar flexion of the toes.

Causes of abnormal reflexes Lower motor neurone lesions cause loss of reflexes associated with the affected nerve. Upper motor neurone lesions result in exaggerated, brisk reflexes due to loss of the modifying influences of upper pathways.

Sudden and sustained stretching of a spastic muscle may result in clonus, which is a sustained rhythmical contraction of the muscle. Ankle clonus is produced by abrupt and continued dorsiflexion of the ankle.

Extensor plantar reflexes (upgoing toes) may be observed:

- during sleep;
- during deep coma from any cause;
- for a short time (up to a few hours) after epileptic convulsions;
- in the first year of life before the corticospinal fibres are fully developed.

In any other circumstances it indicates an organic lesion of the opposite cerebral cortex or the corticospinal tract of the same side (i.e. an upper motor neurone lesion).

Involuntary movements

Examination Look for abnormal movements including fasciculation (twitching), tremor, choreiform movements (non-repetitive, involuntary, abrupt and jerky) and athetoid movements (slow-moving and writhing, particularly affecting the distal parts of limbs).

Causes Muscles that are undergoing denervation develop spontaneous irregular contractions of separate motor units, visible as fasciculations.

A fine tremor may be familial or a feature of anxiety, thyrotoxicosis, alcoholism or excessive caffeine consumption.

Parkinson's disease (see pp. 195–6) produces a slow, coarse, 'pill-rolling' tremor of the fingers, which is reduced by voluntary movements.

In cerebellar disease a tremor develops on purposeful movement (intention tremor) but is usually absent at rest.

A 'flapping' tremor of the outstretched hands occurs in liver failure and hypercapnia (CO_2 retention).

Choreiform and athetoid movements occur with lesions of the extrapyramidal system.

Features distinguishing a lower motor neurone lesion from an upper one are shown in Table 2.3, p. 136.

Sensory system

Anatomy The pathway of sensory fibres from the posterior horn ganglion to the sensory cortex depends on the type of sensation they carry (Fig. 2.29, p. 137; Anatomy box 12, p. 136).

Anatomy box 12
Sensory system

Proprioception (joint position sense), fine touch, vibration and muscle and tendon sensation
Carried in the dorsal column to the nucleus gracilis (legs) and nucleus cuneatus (arms) in the medulla
Cross in the medulla and then radiate to the thalamus, reticular formation, and sensory cortex

Light touch and pressure fibres
Mostly ascend six to eight segments in the dorsal column and then cross to run in the ventral spinothalamic tract

Pain and temperature fibres
Cross at the level they enter the cord to run in the lateral spinothalamic tract

Table 2.3 Features distinguishing a lower motor neurone lesion from an upper motor neurone lesion

	Upper motor neurone	Lower motor neurone
Wasting	Absent or mild	Marked
Fasciculation	Absent	May be present
Tone	Usually increased (spasticity)	Decreased or absent
Power	Reduced	Reduced
Reflexes	Brisk	Absent

To test sensation accurately it is essential to explain the testing procedure to the patient. Test all patients for:
- light touch sensation;
- pain sensation;
- vibration sensation;
- position sensation.
  If sensory abnormalities are detected, test:
- temperature sensation using tubes containing warm and cold water;
- deep pain sensation by squeezing muscles or tendons.

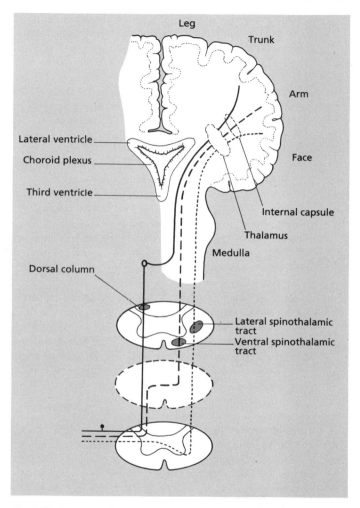

Fig. 2.29 Sensory pathways. ——, Proprioception, light touch, vibration, muscle and tendon sensation; − − −, light touch, pressure; ----, pain, temperature.

Use cotton wool to test *light touch sensation* and pin-prick to test *pain sensation* — both are familiar sensations to the patient. Ask the patient to close their eyes and say whether they feel the cotton wool or a pin-prick. Compare each side in turn and interchange and alter the sensations to ensure that they are actually recognized. For example test with 'the hidden pin' — hold the pin to the pulp of your forefinger with your thumb and introduce it as a stimulus unexpectedly. Ask the patient to tell you whether the stimulus is a 'finger' or a 'finger with a pin'.

NB: Always use a sterile pin for each patient to prevent the very small risk of cross-infection (hepatitis, AIDS).

To test *vibration sensation* ensure that the patient recognizes vibration by placing the tuning fork on the sternum. Then place the vibrating tuning fork on bony prominences on the patient, and ask the patient whether they can feel the vibration. Start distally on the medial malleolus or styloid process and work proximally, comparing right with left and with yourself.

To test *position sensation* hold the patient's big toe or finger by its sides (holding the top or bottom introduces touch sensation) as the patient watches. Move the toe or finger away from the patient explaining 'this is down', and towards the patient explaining 'this is up'. Then ask the patient to close their eyes and say whether the toe or finger is moved up or down as you move it several times. Start with large movements and then gradually make them smaller.

Sensory dermatomes (the area of skin supplied by a particular sensory nerve root) are shown in Fig. 2.30.

Causes of sensory loss The pattern of sensory loss observed in the limbs depends on the site of any lesion.

Peripheral sensory neuropathy tends to cause a symmetrical and initially distal (glove and stocking) loss of sensation, which is more marked in the lower limbs. It is a feature of diabetes mellitus, chronic renal failure, carcinomatous neuropathy, vitamin B_{12} deficiency and treatment with certain drugs.

Spinal cord lesions tend to give rise to a 'sensory level' with loss of sensation at and below the dermatome corresponding with the segmental level of the cord lesion. If not all of the sensory tracts are involved there may be 'dissociated sensory

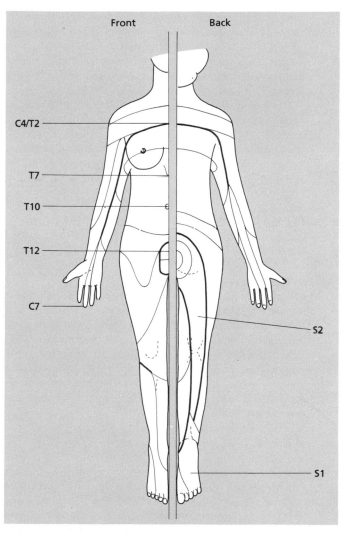

Fig. 2.30 Sensory dermatomes with key points to remember.

loss' with diminution only of the sensation carried by the tracts involved. In the Brown–Séquard syndrome (hemisection of the cord) there is corticospinal (pyramidal) and posterior column (vibration and position sense) loss on the same side and spinothalamic (pain and temperature) loss on the opposite side.

Cerebral lesions cause disturbed sensation of the face and body on the opposite side to the lesion. There may be hemianaesthesia (internal capsule lesions), unpleasant paraesthesia (thalamic lesions) or loss of recognition of objects by touch (astereognosis) and sensory discrimination (parietal cortical lesions).

EXAMINATION OF THE LOCOMOTOR SYSTEM

Joints (Examination box 8, p. 141)

'Ask, look, feel, move'

Joints that are painful or have been noted to be abnormal during the preceding examination should be examined in more detail. Always ask the patient whether the abnormal joint is painful before examining it and do not move any joint beyond the point of pain. Inspect the joint and assess its range of movement (active and passive), comparing it with the other side.

Gout is excruciatingly painful and many patients will be reluctant to let anyone near the affected joint, let alone move it.

Examination Diseased joints are:

- stiff with limited movement;
- painful;
- swollen;
- tender to pressure.

Early morning stiffness describes joint stiffness present on waking and settling after 30 minutes to 1 hour. It is a typical feature of inflammatory arthritis, such as rheumatoid arthritis, and its seronegative (i.e. rheumatoid factor-negative) variants, such as psoriatic arthritis, Reiter's disease and sacroiliitis (ankylosing spondylitis).

Examination box 8
Normal joint movement (range in degrees)

Spine
Flexion (45)
Extension (45)
Lateral bending (45)
Rotation (70)
Sacroiliac joint tenderness is elicited by firm pressure of the palm
  downwards onto the sacrum as the patient lies face down

Shoulder
Flexion (90)
Extension (65)
Adduction (180)
Internal rotation (90)
External rotation (60)

Elbow
Flexion (150)
Pronation (80)
Supination (90)

Wrist
Flexion (praying position, 75)
Extension (reverse praying position, 70)
Ulnar deviation (30), radial deviation (20)
Metacarpophalangeal joints — test grip

Hip joint
Flexion (115)
Extension (30)
Adduction (45)
Abduction (50)
Internal rotation (45)
External rotation (45)

Knee joint
Flexion (135)
Extension (5 hyperextension)

Ankle (a pure hinge joint)
Dorsiflexion (20)
Plantarflexion (50)

Look Examine painful joints for:
- swelling of surrounding soft tissue or because of a joint effusion;
- deformity — e.g. ulnar deviation of the wrist in chronic rheumatoid arthritis, genu varum (knock knees), genu valgus (bow legs), hallux valgus (osteoarthritis causing a bunion at the first metatarsophalangeal joint).
- discoloration — redness of acute inflammation and infection;
- muscle wasting.

Feel Feel for any tenderness or increase in temperature. It may be difficult to differentiate an effusion of synovial fluid in the knee from synovial thickening, which occurs in inflammatory arthritis. Confirmatory signs of an effusion are the fluid bulge sign and the patella tap.

To elicit the fluid bulge sign fill the joint with fluid by exerting pressure on the suprapatellar region when the leg is relaxed and straight. Then, firmly and smoothly stroke each side of the patella alternately. If fluid is present this will move fluid from one side of the joint to the other and the joint will bulge on the opposite side.

To elicit the patella tap fill the joint as described for the fluid bulge sign and push the patella down gently but firmly. If fluid is present it will produce a palpable 'tap' when the patella contacts the femur beneath.

Sacroiliac joint tenderness is elicited by firm pressure of the palm downwards onto the sacrum as the patient lies face down.

Move Ask the patient to demonstrate the joint's range of active movements. They will limit these if painful. Then compare the range of passive movements, taking care not to cause any distress.

Test joint mobility within the limits of pain. The normal range can be easily assessed by examining your own or a colleague's joints.

To assess metacarpophalangeal joint function, test grip.

Joint stability at the knee depends on stable cruciate ligaments. To test the ligaments bend the patient's leg and sit on their foot, and attempt to move the tibia backward and forward on the femur. Excess movement suggests instability.

To test the lateral ligaments hold the patient's femur down

flat. Then grasp the tibia gently and firmly and attempt to move it medially and laterally at the knee.

Arthritis

Systemic features

Inflammatory arthritis (e.g. rheumatoid arthritis) is part of a generalized disease involving all systems. The joints are often symmetrically involved. Organs particularly involved are the eyes and the skin.

Look at the skin for:
- tophi of gout — found around joints and on the cartilage of the ears;
- subcutaneous nodules at the elbow in rheumatoid arthritis;
- tight skin and/or superficial calcification of the fingers in scleroderma;
- thimble pitting of nails (Fig. 2.1) and psoriasis, usually at the elbow, in psoriatic arthritis;
- red or brown nailfold infarcts (Fig. 2.1) due to vasculitis in rheumatoid arthritis;
- superficial redness over an infected or gouty joint.

Look at the eyes for:
- dryness (and dry mouth from decreased saliva) in Sjögren's disease;
- conjunctivitis of Reiter's disease;
- iritis of ankylosing spondylitis;
- scleritis of rheumatoid arthritis.

Common causes of arthritis are:
- osteoarthritis;
- rheumatoid arthritis;
- gout.

Osteoarthritis

Osteoarthritis is an asymmetrical arthritis. It often involves weight-bearing joints — commonly the hip, and also the terminal interphalangeal joints of the hands. It is most commonly seen in the elderly, who may present with nodules (see p. 54) around the terminal interphalangeal joints. The following are three tests used to detect hip disease in osteoarthritis.

The Trendelenburg test Normally standing on one leg causes the pelvis on the other side to tilt upward to ensure balance (try it yourself). When balancing on an osteoarthritic hip that side of the pelvis tilts downward because of loss of purchase for the pelvifemoral muscles around the diseased joint.

True shortening of the leg The distance between the anterior superior iliac spine and the medial malleolus is shorter on the osteoarthritic side because of reduced joint space.

Fixed flexion When testing full flexion in the normal leg, the other osteoarthritic hip lifts off the couch as the pelvis rolls upward to compensate for the lack of natural extension of the femur on the diseased side.

Rheumatoid arthritis

Rheumatoid arthritis is usually symmetrical. It predominantly affects the hands, causing swelling of the proximal finger joints and ulnar deviation of the fingers, and also the wrists, with muscle wasting around affected joints. Rheumatoid nodules may be present over the lower ulnar at the elbows.

In severe long-standing rheumatoid disease (and also disabling neurological disease), disability may be severe and is classified into four grades: (i) complete independence — no support needed; (ii) independent with support, such as adapted and special appliances at work and home; (iii) partially dependent, requiring assistance for complex movement such as bathing and dressing; and (iv) totally dependent, being confined to a wheelchair or bed.

Gout

Gout may affect any joint, but commonly involves the metatarsophalangeal joint of the big toe, which becomes red, hot, shiny and tender. Tophi (white, chalky deposits of uric acid crystals) may develop over joints and around the ears.

Septic infected arthritis must be considered in the diagnosis of any acutely inflamed joint.

Lumps

When examining any lump, note:
- site;

- shape;
- consistency;
- fixation;
- fluctuation and transillumination (? fluid-filled);
- pulsation and auscultation (? vascular);

and examine local lymph nodes for enlargement due to spread of malignancy or infection.

Lumps in the skin
Sebaceous cyst

Age Rare before adolescence.

Site Any except soles of feet and palms of hands (lack sebaceous glands). Common on scalp.

Clinical features Tense, spherical, non-tender lumps with normal overlying skin (unless infected, usually following trauma, when become tender, warm and red).

Lipoma

Age Any.

Site Any; common in subcutaneous tissues of upper limbs.

Clinical features Smooth, lobulated, mobile lump with normal overlying skin.

Malignant melanoma

Malignant change in a mole or pigmented naevus.

Age Any, but rare before puberty.

Clinical features Malignant change in a mole or pigmented naevus is suggested by:
- increase in size, shape or thickness;
- itching;
- change in colour;
- bleeding;
- evidence of distant spread — lymphadenopathy, nodules around primary lesion (satellite nodules).

Basal cell carcinoma

Age Incidence increases with age (related to duration of ultra-violet (UV) light exposure).

Site Common on face.

Clinical features Slow-growing nodule or ulcer with raised, rolled edge. May bleed and become infected. Does not metastasize so local lymph nodes should not be enlarged unless infected.

Squamous cell carcinoma

Age Increases with age (UV light exposure).

Site Sun-exposed skin.

Clinical features Red-brown nodule which may ulcerate. Grows more rapidly than basal cell carcinoma. Local lymphadenopathy may occur as a result of spread or infection.

Keratoacanthoma

Self-limiting overgrowth of hair follicle cells which regresses spontaneously. May be mistaken for squamous cell carcinoma but has usually regressed within 2−3 months.

Lumps in the neck (Fig. 2.4)

Common causes of lumps

Enlarged thyroid Mass on one or both sides of thyroid that moves on swallowing. Examine: trachea for displacement; draining lymph nodes in anterior triangle of neck for signs of hypo- or hyperthyroidism.

Branchial cyst Remnant of second branchial arch. Soft swelling which bulges forward from beneath the anterior border of the sternomastoid in the carotid triangle.

Lymph nodes Most commonly due to: infection (e.g. TB, local sepsis, glandular fever, CMV); malignancy (lymphoma or metastatic).

Skin Lipoma, sebaceous cyst.

Less common causes

Salivary gland Tumours or infection (mumps or bacterial), Sjögren's syndrome (p. 199).

Pharyngeal pouch

Carotid artery aneurysm

Breast lumps

Any lump in the breast should be regarded as potentially malignant and subjected to excision biopsy (with the exception of a cyst which disappears completely on aspiration).

Common causes are:

- carcinoma;
- 'chronic mastitis' (with or without cysts);
- fibroadenoma.

Features which suggest malignancy are:

- hard, non-tender, irregular lump;
- fixation to the skin;
- orange peel appearance of the skin (*peau d'orange*) due to lymphatic obstruction;
- palpable axillary lymph nodes.

Fibroadenomas are highly mobile, smooth, firm benign tumours ('breast mice').

Groin lumps

The commonest cause of a lump in the groin is a hernia. Lumps may also arise from:

- lymph nodes;
- skin — lipoma;
- vessels — varicosity of the saphenous vein (saphena varix) or aneurysm of femoral artery;
- genitalia — spermatocoele of the cord or ectopic testis;
- muscle — psoas abscess.

Examination box 9
Method for examining the whole patient

First
Greet the patient
Examine the hands
Feel the pulse
Take the blood pressure

Head and neck
Look at facial appearance, conjunctivae
Examine mouth and pharynx
Feel for lymph nodes in the neck

Continued overleaf

Examination box 9 *Contd*

Heart and lungs

Examine the internal and external jugular veins

Ensure the trachea is central

Feel for the left ventricle apex and right ventricle hypertrophy and cardiac thrills

Listen to the heart — apex, parasternal

From the front: observe and palpate chest movements; percuss the lungs, listen to the lungs

Sit the patient forward and repeat test for movements, percussion, breath sounds

Abdomen

Observe during quiet breathing

Palpate gently for masses and to exclude tenderness

Examine:

    for enlarged organs (liver, spleen, kidneys)

    right and left iliac fossae (colonic masses)

    the mid-line — stomach in epigastrium, umbilical region

    suprapubically for bladder uterus and ovaries

    for herniae and inguinal nodes

    external genitalia

Perform rectal (and if indicated vaginal) examination

Nervous system

Test cranial nerves

Upper limbs

Look for bone and joint deformity, inflammation, muscle wasting

Examine the joints

Examine power, posture, tone coordination, reflexes

Lower limbs

Look for bone and joint deformity, inflammation, muscle wasting

Look at feet for hair (absent if ischaemic) and infection

Feel feet for temperature — compare right and left

Examine joints

Examine power, posture, tone, coordination, reflexes, Romberg's test, gait and heel–toe walking

SUMMARY

A suggested method for examining the whole patient is shown in Examination box 9 on pp. 147–8. This method is commonly used by family doctors and hospital physicians. It has been found to be the most convenient because it starts with the hands and ends with the feet, and allows for completeness with economy of effort by both the doctor and the patient.

2

3 Diseases

3

3

RESPIRATORY DISEASES

Upper respiratory diseases

Common cold

Predisposing factors Enclosed gatherings.

Aetiology More than 150 viruses, e.g. adeno virus, rhino virus, entero virus (Coxsackie virus and echo virus), influenza, respiratory syncytial virus (RSV).

Symptoms

Fever (may be afebrile).

Runny nose and sneeze.

Sore throat and painful swallowing.

Signs Red throat of pharyngitis.

Management Symptomatic with analgesia (paracetamol or aspirin — avoid aspirin in children under 12 (p. 154)).

Steam inhalation for tracheitis and bronchitis.

Nasal decongestants.

Complications Predisposes to secondary bacterial infection causing sinusitis and otitis media.

Pharyngitis and tonsillitis

Aetiology Common cold viruses (90%) and occasionally Epstein–Barr (EB) virus of glandular fever.

Haemolytic *Streptococcus* (Lancefield group A; 5%).

Symptoms

Sore throat.

Pain on swallowing.

Signs Red pharynx and enlarged red tonsils.

Investigations Throat swab for bacterial culture (for haemolytic *Streptococcus*).

Blood for EB virus antibodies if glandular fever suspected (monospot test gives rapid and reliable answer — positive in 90% of cases).

Treatment Symptomatic as for colds with aspirin or paracetamol.

Penicillin for haemolytic streptococcal infection.

Quinsy

Peritonsillar bacterial abscess secondary to streptococcal

pharyngitis — unilateral but may be confused with severe glandular fever. Can cause obstruction to swallowing and airway and requires surgical drainage.

Hoarseness

Hoarseness is a common feature of upper tract infections which often involve the larynx. In the absence of other features of infection, hoarseness persisting for more than 2−3 weeks suggests disease of the vocal cords (e.g. singer's nodule or laryngeal carcinoma) and expert ear−nose−throat (ENT) advice is needed.

Glandular fever (infectious mononucleosis)

Aetiology EB virus.

Symptoms

Fever.

Muscle aches.

Sore throat.

Painful enlargement of neck lymph nodes.

Rash.

Signs Red enlarged tonsils and grey surface exudate (occasionally sufficient to obstruct swallowing and even breathing).

Large tender cervical glands.

Splenomegaly.

Diffuse macular (flat)/papular (slightly raised) red skin rash.

Investigations

White blood cells (WBC) increased with 'glandular fever' cells seen on film (atypical mononuclear cells with granular nuclei and foamy cytoplasm).

Monospot positive.

Antibodies present to EB virus.

Platelet count may be reduced.

Liver enzymes may be raised (due to associated hepatitis).

Management Symptomatic with simple analgesics (paracetamol, aspirin).

Prednisolone to reduce acute inflammation and tonsillar swelling if there is obstruction to swallowing or breathing.

NB: Diphtheria (in tropics and unimmunized) has similar appearance.

Sinusitis

Aetiology Viral or bacterial infection (*Haemophilus influenzae* or *Streptococcus pneumoniae* secondary to upper tract virus infection).

Symptoms

Fever — hot and cold shivers (features of a bacterial abscess).

Pain over sinuses (usually maxillary) and upper jaws.

Mucopurulent nasal discharge.

Management Reduce fever and pain with aspirin, or pain with paracetamol.

Nasal decongestants if symptoms mild.

Antibiotics (amoxycillin or Augmentin — amoxycillin plus clavulinic acid — which will also attack anaerobes) for suspected bacterial infections.

Acute otitis media

This is usually seen in children under 3–4 years old.

Aetiology Bacterial infection (*Streptococcus pneumoniae* or *Haemophilus influenzae*, haemolytic *Streptococcus*) often secondary to upper respiratory tract infection.

Symptoms

Severe earache and hearing loss.

Fever and shivers (symptoms of abscess formation).

Signs Tympanic membrane (ear drum) red and bulging.

Complications Rupture of drum, spread of infection to mastoid, brain (meningitis, abscess, venous sinus thrombosis).

Management Analgesia with paracetamol. Do not give aspirin to children under 12 years — possible link with encephalitis, fatty liver infiltration and hypoglycaemia of Reye's syndrome.

Antibiotics (amoxycillin) oral if mild, intravenous if severe.

Myringotomy (incision into tympanic membrane) may be required to drain pus and prevent rupture — incisions heal better than ruptures.

Acute laryngeal obstruction
Foreign bodies

The commonest foreign bodies are fish bones, which cause choking, and meat lumps aspirated unchewed (particularly if the pharyngeal reflexes are suppressed by alcohol). Obstruction is rarely complete.

Management Reassure patient and encourage to breathe through nose.

Inspect throat, depressing tongue with spatula or spoon, and attempt removal with tweezers if easily seen and reached.

Turn head down, or upside down if a child, and hit in the back.

If respiration seriously or progressively embarrassed, attempt Heimlich manoeuvre — grasp the patient from behind and exert sudden pressure in the epigastrium directed upward through the diaphragm (a modified bear hug).

In hospital seek ENT or anaesthetic expert advice.

NB: Forcing food further down is more dangerous. Do not attempt removal of foreign bodies unless easy.

Acute anaphylaxis (acute angio-oedema)

Part of hypersensitivity reaction to bee-sting, vaccines (live, e.g. yellow fever), iodine (in X-ray contrast media).

Signs Flushing of skin, itching and urticaria (red raised weals).

Severe attacks progress to wheezing with swelling of lips and tongue and finally laryngeal obstruction.

Management Adrenaline 0.5–1.0 ml of 1/1000 strength, intramuscularly (IM). Then repeat every 15 minutes according to pulse and blood pressure until improvement is seen.

NB: Steroids and antihistamines can also be given but take too long to act in acute anaphylaxis.

Hydrocortisone 200–400 mg intravenously (IV), then as an infusion for 10–12 hours.

Lower respiratory diseases

Acute bronchitis

Predisposing factors Smoking, atmospheric pollution.

Aetiology Acute virus, *Mycoplasma* or bacterial (*Streptococcus pneumoniae*, *Haemophilus influenzae*) infection.

Symptoms

Cough.

Sputum — yellow and/or green.

Dyspnoea and wheeze.

Fever.

Signs
Dyspnoea at rest.
Wheezing.
Coarse inspiratory and expiratory crackles at lung bases.

Investigations Sputum for Gram-stain and culture if unwell. Lung function tests (p. 310) show both reduced peak flow rate (PFR) (obstructive defect) and reduced forced expiratory volume in 1 second (FEV_1) during attack.

NB: Lung function often normal between attacks. Chest X-ray (CXR) usually normal.

Management Stop smoking.

Bronchodilators for wheeze (β_2-adrenoreceptor agonists — salbutamol, terbutaline).

Antibiotics (amoxycillin or trimethoprim for *Streptococcus pneumoniae* and *Haemophilus influenzae*).

Chronic bronchitis

Repeated attacks of acute bronchitis leading eventually to non-reversible lung disease with persistent reduction in measures of lung function. (Medical Research Council (MRC) definition = daily cough and sputum for 3 months in at least 2 consecutive years).

Predisposing factors Smoking, pollution. Exacerbated by infection.

Symptoms
Cough and morning sputum — persistent sputum production.
Dyspnoea — breathlessness becomes progressively worse.
Wheezing with acute exacerbations.

Signs
Early disease Dyspnoea with wheeze in acute episodes.
Coarse crackles at lung bases.
Late disease Persistent dyspnoea with reduced effort tolerance.
Hyperinflated 'barrel' chest of air-trapping.
Raised jugular venous pulse (JVP), liver enlargement and ankle oedema of right heart failure (secondary to pulmonary hypertension).

Investigation
CXR Normal early. Late: overinflation of lungs with low flat diaphragms.

Lung function Reduced PFR, reduced FEV_1 and forced vital capacity (FVC). FEV_1/FVC ratio also reduced.

Arterial gases Normal early. Later reduced partial pressure of arterial oxygen (PaO_2) and increased partial pressure of arterial carbon dioxide ($PaCO_2$) and decreased pH.

Management Stop smoking.

Bronchodilators if airways outflow obstruction reversible (assess by measuring PFR before and after bronchodilator).

Antibiotics for acute infections (amoxycillin or trimethoprim).

For late disease Steroids may partially relieve airways obstruction (confirm response by lung function tests before giving long-term).

Physiotherapy.

Oxygen (controlled at 24–28%) – long-term domiciliary oxygen helps to prevent hospital admission.

Treat right heart failure with diuretics.

Asthma (see p. 229 for treatment of severe asthma)

Predisposing factors

External allergens – pollen, animal fur, house mite, aspirin.

Exercise.

Cold atmosphere.

Symptoms Episodic cough, dyspnoea and usually wheeze.

Severe attacks Persistent and progressive dyspnoea, chest tightness and wheeze.

Signs

Dyspnoea.

Expiratory and inspiratory wheezes.

Severe attacks (status asthmaticus) Persistent severe dyspnoea – may be too breathless to speak and wheeze may be absent if very little air is moving in airways.

Cyanosis.

Tachycardia and pulsus paradoxus.

NB: Sudden death may occur.

Investigations CXR to exclude pneumothorax and infection.

Lung function – mild attacks Reduced PFR and FEV_1. PFR is usually worse in the morning.

Lung function – severe attacks Unable to use peak flow meter or markedly reduced (less than 100 litres/min).

Arterial gases Reduced PaO_2 (feature of early respiratory failure).

Increased $PaCO_2$ and decreased pH in very severe cases.

Management

Prevention Regular inhalation with β_2 agonist bronchodilators (salbutamol, terbutaline).

Steroid inhalation (Becotide) if β_2 agonists insufficient.

Acute attacks (p. 229)

Consider severe if persists for more than 2–4 hours.

Continuous oxygen at high concentration (use nasal cannulae to deliver up to 100%).

Beta$_2$ agonists by nebulizer.

IV fluids.

IV steroids.

Consider artificial ventilation for progressive respiratory failure (rising or raised $PaCO_2$).

Pneumonia

Infection within the lung tissue.

Classification *Lobar* – affecting one lobe of one lung only. Usually caused by *Streptococcus pneumoniae* (pneumococcal pneumonia).

Bronchopneumonia – affects different parts of different lobes of both lungs. May be bacterial, mycoplasmal or viral.

Lobar pneumonia

Aetiology *Streptococcus pneumoniae* infection.

Symptoms

Acute and sudden onset of fever.

Rigors (shaking with hot and cold chills).

Rusty (blood-stained) sputum.

Signs

Dyspnoea.

Cyanosis if severe.

Consolidation with bronchial breathing over affected lobe.

Investigations

Sputum for Gram-stain to confirm bacterium.

Blood for culture (positive in 50% of cases).

CXR shows consolidation in one lobe with air bronchogram

(the airways are outlined in black within the white consolidated lung).

NB: Loss of lung volume within the consolidated lung suggests proximal obstruction, e.g. carcinoma of bronchus.

Management

Oxygen in high concentration.

Physiotherapy.

Penicillin 1.2 g IV daily in four divided doses.

Bronchopneumonia

Aetiology

- Viral — measles, chickenpox, RSV*, influenza;
- mycoplasma — *Mycoplasma pneumoniae**;
- bacterial — *Streptococcus**, *Pneumococcus*, *Legionella pneumophilia* (Legionnaire's disease), *Staphylococcus aureus*, *Klebsiella pneumoniae*, psittacosis, tuberculosis (TB) (common in developing world).

NB: Immunosuppressed patients, i.e. those on steroids, azathioprine or with acquired immunodeficiency syndrome (AIDS) develop opportunistic lung infections with viruses (cytomegalovirus (CMV), herpes zoster), bacteria (TB) and fungi (*Monilia* and *Aspergillus*).

Symptoms

Fever and rigors.

Cough.

Purulent sputum.

Signs

Dyspnoea.

Cyanosis.

Signs of consolidation over affected parts of lungs.

Investigations

Sputum for Gram-stain.

Blood for culture. Serial blood samples to look for rising antibody titres.

CXR shows patchy areas of consolidation with air bronchogram(s).

Management As lobar pneumonia.

Antibiotics as guided by Gram-stain — if not helpful, start with erythromycin to cover likely bacteria (asterisked above).

* Denotes most common.

Bronchial carcinoma

This causes 20% of cancer deaths in men, 5% in women annually.

Aetiology

Cigarette smoking (squamous and oat cell carcinoma).

Asbestos exposure.

Symptoms

Often none — detected on CXR.

Cough.

Haemoptysis.

Anorexia and weight loss.

Dyspnoea if sufficient lung collapsed.

Pleuritic pain if pleura involved.

Bone pain if bony metastases.

Epileptic fits if cerebral metastases.

Signs

Pulmonary

Dyspnoea.

Pleural effusion.

Collapsed lung if large airway obstructed.

Non-pulmonary Metastatic tumour deposits give:

- lymph node enlargement (neck and supraclavicular);
- liver enlargement;
- focal neurological signs (cerebral involvement);
- atrial fibrillation (pericardial involvement);
  Non-metastatic manifestations are:
- clubbing of nails;
- dementia and cerebellar ataxia;
- dermatomyositis;
- ectopic hormone production (adenocorticotrophic hormone (ACTH), parathyroid hormone, antidiuretic hormone (ADH), prolactin).

Investigations

Blood count for anaemia and raised erythrocyte sedimentation rate (ESR) and C-reactive protein (CRP) (p. 265).

Liver function tests (liver metastases).

Calcium (bony metastases or ectopic parathyroid hormone production).

CXR for hilar or peripheral rounded lesion, pulmonary collapse, pleural effusion.

Computed tomography (CT) scan to define tumour and spread locally and to liver and adrenals. Isotope bone scan if bony metastases suspected.

Sputum for cytology to detect tumour cells.

Bronchoscopy with biopsy.

Management Surgery if removable — CT scan to determine if tumour localized and absence of secondary spread (15–20% are resectable, 30% of these survive 5 years).

Radiotherapy for bone pain and superior vena caval (SVC) obstruction.

Chemotherapy remains of little value except squamous cell carcinoma (SCC).

Diphosphonates for bone pain.

Sarcoid

Aetiology Unknown. Possibly a TB variant as typical histology shows granuloma with giant cells but without caseation.

Symptoms

Tiredness and fever.

Erythema nodosum.

Arthralgia — usually ankles and knees.

Painful red eyes.

Signs

Erythema nodosum.

Acute iritis.

There are usually no chest signs.

NB: Chronic sarcoid is rare and presents with progressive dyspnoea over months or years from slowly progressive fibrosis of alveolar tissue.

NB: 'Non-pulmonary' sarcoid is rare and affects:

- skin (10%) (erythema nodosum);
- lymph nodes (30%) (generalized lymphadenopathy);
- liver and spleen (10%) (enlargement);
- eyes (10%) (uveitis);
- nervous system, including epilepsy;
- bones (cysts);
- endocrine system (diabetes insipidus).

Investigations (of pulmonary sarcoid)

CXR for symmetrical enlargement of hilar lymph nodes.

Blood for raised ESR and raised CRP.

Blood for raised calcium (increased 1,25 dihydroxy vitamin D).

Kveim test (intradermal injection of standard sarcoid tissue) may be positive but takes 4−6 weeks and risks transmission of infection.

Tuberculosis

See infections, pp. 222−3.

Pneumothorax (air within pleural space)

Aetiology Cause usually unknown (spontaneous pneumothorax) and presumed to follow rupture of a small bulla on pleural surface. Ectomorphs (tall, thin people).

Associated with asthma, TB.

Symptoms

Sudden acute stabbing pleural pain and dyspnoea.

Progressive dyspnoea if pleural air under 'tension' (may cause rapid death if not relieved − for treatment see p. 229).

Signs May be none detectable. Classical signs are:

- chest movement on affected side reduced;
- percussion hyperresonant;
- breath sounds reduced;
- vocal resonance reduced;
- tactile fremitus reduced.

NB: In tension pneumothorax there is also:

- rapid and progressive dyspnoea;
- tracheal deviation − away from affected side.

Investigations CXR to detect pneumothorax and follow progress (needs draining if greater than 50% of one side affected) or presence of early tension (tracheal deviation).

Most small pneumothoraces resolve spontaneously.

Management Insert intercostal drain if there is loss of more than 50% of lung volume.

Consider aspiration.

Insert intercostal drain *urgently* if tension present.

Cystic fibrosis

Inherited disorder of exocrine glands. Abnormal viscous secretions in lungs, pancreas. Lungs physiologically normal at birth, damaged by repeated childhood infections.

Aetiology Autosomal recessive disorder. Incidence 1 : 2000; carrier rate 1 : 20.

Symptoms

Failure to thrive as infant.

Recurrent bacterial chest infections progressing to bronchiectasis.

Malabsorption.

Signs

Stunted growth.

Clubbing.

Coarse crackles in chest.

Diagnosis

Sweat sodium > 70 mM.

Treatment

Antibiotics for chest infections.

Physiotherapy.

Postural drainage.

Pancreatic supplements with food.

Fibrosing alveolitis

Aetiology Unknown in most cases (cryptogenic); may be associated with connective tissue disease (e.g. systemic lupus erythematosus (SLE)).

Symptoms

Progressive dyspnoea.

Unproductive cough.

Signs

Mid and late inspiratory crackles in lower zones.

Finger clubbing.

Investigations

CXR — reticular shadowing. Shrinking of lungs with elevation of diaphragms.

Lung function — low FEV_1, FVC and transfer factor.

Blood gases (p. 310).

Management Steroids beneficial in some cases.

Oxygen.

CARDIOVASCULAR DISEASES

Angina

Aetiology

Cigarette smoking.
Hypertension.
Hyperlipidaemia.
Obesity.

Precipitating factors

Exercise.
Cold weather.
Heavy meal.
Aortic stenosis.
Paroxysmal tachycardia.
Severe anaemia.
Myxoedema.

Symptoms

Central tight chest pain on exertion and particularly in cold weather.
The pain radiates to the throat, jaw and arms.
Relieved by rest and glyceryl trinitrate.

Signs There are usually no abnormal heart signs if uncomplicated.

Complications

Sudden death (40%), usually from acute rhythm change (ventricular fibrillation (VF) or ventricular tachycardia (VT)) cardiovascular shock.
Myocardial infarction (below).
Cardiac failure — poor cardiac output (below).
Arrhythmias.

Investigations

Blood count for anaemia and thyroid function.
CXR for heart size and outline of cardiac chambers.
Electrocardiogram (ECG) for ischaemic changes seen in ST segments but normal in uncomplicated angina.
Treadmill stress test.
Coronary angiography if angina on minimal exertion or ischaemic ECG during treadmill exercise.

Management

Lose weight.

Dress warmly in cold weather.

Glyceryl trinitrate sublingually for pain or before exertion known to induce pain, e.g. housework, climbing inclines.

Calcium channel blockers.

Beta-blockers.

Other nitrates.

Treat hypertension and lipids, hypothyroidism, aortic valve disorders, arrhythmias, anaemia.

Coronary angioplasty or coronary artery bypass graft (CABG) if treatable lesion on angiography.

Myocardial infarction

Aetiology Death of heart muscle, usually due to thrombus (clot) formation in a narrowed, atheromatous artery. Rarer causes (consider if no risk factors present) include coronary artery embolus and coronary artery vasculitis.

Symptoms

Central tight pain usually greater than half an hour's duration.

Not relieved by rest or glyceryl trinitrate.

Cold sweat from hypotension.

Dyspnoea from early left ventricular failure (LVF).

Palpitation if rhythm change.

Signs

None if uncomplicated.

Hypotension with pallor and cold sweat, often secondary to rhythm change.

Cardiac failure — dyspnoea on rest with fine bilateral crackles at lung bases (see also acute pulmonary oedema, p. 230).

Bradycardia or tachycardia, which may be regular (sinus or atrioventricular (AV) node initiated) or irregular (atrial fibrillation or flutter: ventricular ectopics).

Complications

Death from cardiac shock (insufficient heart muscle or rhythm change) or rupture of the myocardium.

LVF.

Papillary muscle dysfunction.

Mitral regurgitation.

Left ventricular aneurysm.

Management

Bed rest.

Oxygen in high concentration.

Pain relief with morphine, diamorphine.

Thrombolysis with streptokinase or anistreplase (APSA) or alteplase (rt-PA).

Aspirin.

Diuretics (frusemide 40–80 mg orally, bumetanide 1–2 mg orally for LV failure; for acute pulmonary oedema give same dose IV stat).

Arrhythmias Treat if causing decreased cardiac output (low blood pressure (BP)) (i.e. leave otherwise uncomplicated sinus tachycardia or bradycardia alone):

- Supraventricular tachycardia (SVT): with (i) carotid massage (massage over one carotid with gentle pressure, using the thumb, to increase vagal tone); (ii) adenosine (3 mg by rapid intravenous injection) controls SVT but not VT; (iii) direct current (DC) cardioversion (delivery of a short high-energy (50–200 J) shock across the heart), using a defibrillator. The defibrillator stores electrical energy, which can be discharged through two paddles, one held over the sternum and the other in the left axilla. Administration of the current causes complete depolarization of the heart, which is followed by a short period of asystole, and usually resumption of normal sinus rhythm. The paddles are coated with electrically conducting jelly or pads to prevent burning of the skin; (iv) verapamil (unless patient has received beta-blocker – risk of asystole).
- Atrial flutter or fibrillation: with DC cardioversion, verapamil, digoxin to slow ventricular rate.
- Complete heart block (ventricular rate 40/minute regular rate): with atropine 0.6 mg IV until insertion of cardiac pacing wire.
- VT: with DC cardioversion; VF: with external cardiorespiratory massage and DC cardioversion.

Cardiomyopathy: hypertrophic and dilated

'Disorder of heart muscle'; classified into hypertrophic and dilated.

Hypertrophic obstructive cardiomyopathy (HOCM)

Asymmetrical hypertrophy of left ventricle, usually familial.

Clinical features Loss of ventricular distensibility and outflow obstruction give rise to the characteristic steeply rising jerky pulse.

Syncope (low cardiac output), dyspnoea and pulmonary oedema may occur. Cardiac arrhythmias and sudden death may also occur.

Investigation Echocardiography shows the ventricular hypertrophy, often with abnormal mitral valve movement.

Management Beta-blockers help relieve the obstruction by increasing peripheral vascular resistance. Anti-arrhythmic treatment may be required — amiodarone is usually effective.

Dilated cardiomyopathy

The common causes of cardiomyopathy (ischaemia, hypertension, valve disease) are usually excluded from the diagnosis.

Aetiology Usually idiopathic, but causes include alcohol, haemochromatosis, sarcoid, drugs (e.g. doxorubicin, cyclophosphamide), amyloid, glycogen storage diseases, connective tissue diseases.

Clinical features Those of cardiac failure (below).

Management As for cardiac failure (below). Treat underlying cause where possible.

Cardiac failure

Pulmonary oedema

Occurs with LVF. The left ventricular muscle pump is inadequate to empty the lungs of intravascular fluid, i.e. pulmonary venous congestion occurs.

Aetiology

Hypertension.

Myocardial ischaemia.

Mitral and aortic valve disease.

Symptoms Progressive dyspnoea on exertion and then at rest, worse lying flat, when blood pools in lungs, causing paroxysmal nocturnal dyspnoea (PND) (waking at night breathless).

Symptoms of right-sided heart failure (see below), which follows LVF.

Signs

Sinus (regular) tachycardia.

Fall of BP and shock are late features.

Displacement of apex if there is hypertrophy or dilatation of the failing left ventricle.

Cardiac triple rhythm (third or fourth sound obvious on auscultation).

Fine bilateral basal crackles at lung bases posteriorly.

Management

Non-acute LVF

Treat underlying causes, i.e. hypertension, valve disorders, abnormal rhythms.

Diuretics (frusemide (oral) 20—80 mg or bumetanide 1—2 mg).

Vasodilators, which take the load off the heart.

Venodilators (e.g. nitrates) reduce the filling pressure of the heart, or 'pre-load', whereas arterial vasodilators (e.g. hydralazine) reduce the resistance the heart pumps against, or 'afterload'. Angiotensin-converting enzyme (ACE) inhibitors cause both arterial and venous vasodilatation.

Acute pulmonary oedema See Emergencies, p. 230.

Right-sided heart failure

Aetiology

Secondary to LVF.

Pulmonary hypertension usually secondary to chronic obstructive airways disease or mitral valve stenosis.

NB: Cor pulmonale is the combination of chronic airways disease and right heart failure.

Symptoms Venous engorgement with ankle oedema (sacral oedema if lying in bed) and later abdominal distension from ascites.

Signs

Raised JVP.

Ankle and/or sacral oedema.

Liver enlargement and tenderness from venous congestion.

Signs of underlying cause.
Management
Treat underlying cause.
Diuretics.

Hypertension

There is no normal BP but the rate of complications, particularly cerebrovascular haemorrhage (stroke) and LVF, increase progressively with increases in diastolic pressure.

Diastolic increases are more serious than systolic and sustained increases more significant than transient elevation of BP.

Pressures below 140 systolic and 90 diastolic (fifth sound) are used as life assurance 'norms'.

Aetiology
Unknown (essential hypertension) (95%).
Alcohol.
Coarctation of the aorta.
Renal disease.
Endocrine disease:
• Cushing's syndrome (increased adrenal corticosteroids).
• Conn's syndrome (increased adrenal mineralocorticoids).
• Phaeochromocytoma (increased adrenaline and noradrenaline from adrenal medulla).
• Acromegaly.
Contraceptive pill.
Eclampsia (toxaemia) of pregnancy.

Symptoms None of BP rise alone.

Signs
Increased BP may be only sign.
Left ventricular hypertrophy.
Hypertensive retinopathy:
• grade I arterial narrowing;
• grade II arteriovenous nipping;
• grade III haemorrhages and exudates;
• grade IV papilloedema (malignant or accelerated hypertension).
NB: Large kidneys of polycystic disease; abdominal bruit of renal artery stenosis; delayed and reduced femoral pulse (radiofemoral delay) of aortic coarctation.

Complications
Cerebral haemorrhage.
LVF.
Myocardial infarction.
Renal failure.
Retinopathy.
Investigations
Blood for renal function and hypokalaemic alkalosis of Cushing's and Conn's syndromes.
Blood or urine for adrenaline and noradrenaline or by-products in young patients.
CXR for left ventricular hypertrophy and rib-notching of coarctation.
ECG for left ventricular hypertrophy (S wave in V_1 plus 'R' in $V_5 > 35$ mm).
Urine for protein, cells and casts.
Management Treat underlying cause. Hypotensive therapy to attain BP of 140/90 — start with one of the following groups:
• low-dose thiazide, e.g. bendrofluazide 2.5 mg daily;
• beta-blocking agents: propranolol, atenolol, metoprolol;
• calcium channel blocker, e.g. nifedipine.

If control not achieved by one agent, try adding member of second group and then adding an ACE inhibitor (enalapril or captopril) but beware if renovascular disease present or suspected, as acute renal failure may be induced.

Accelerated hypertension (see Emergencies, p. 230).

Valvular heart disease
Symptoms usually follow complications of left- (pp. 167–8) or right-sided heart failure (pp. 168–9).
Signs are shown in Fig. 2.7 (p. 72).

Infective endocarditis
Aetiology Infection on abnormal (rheumatic, congenital or calcified) valves or other structural abnormalities (e.g. septal defects, patent ductus arteriosus) is usually insidious and bacterial in origin (subacute bacterial endocarditis). *Streptococcus viridans* (commensal in mouth, bacteraemia follows dental manipulation) is the commonest organism.

Other organisms include: *Staphylococcus aureus* and *S. albus*, *Streptococcus faecalis*, *Coxiella burnetii* (*Rickettsia*-like organism which causes Q fever) and fungi (*Candida*, aspergilli). Rarely it complicates an acute septicaemia (acute endocarditis).

Clinical features

General Lethargy, malaise, weight loss, fever, arthralgia, anaemia. Clubbing and splenomegaly are late signs.

Cardiac Changing murmurs (examine the patient daily). Signs of an underlying cardiac lesion may not be present.

Embolic Large emboli to brain or other viscera.

Splinter haemorrhages, Osler's nodes (painful haemorrhagic lesions in the fingertips) and Roth's spots (retinal haemorrhages) are thought to represent either 'microemboli' or vasculitis (inflammation of small blood vessels).

Haematuria may result from emboli to the kidneys or glomerulonephritis.

Investigation Repeat blood cultures (at least three) before starting treatment. The ESR is usually raised; the white cell count may be raised, normal or low. Check renal function and mid-stream urine (MSU) for microscopic haematuria; CXR, ECG and echocardiogram for cardiac abnormalities.

Management

Prophylaxis Patients with cardiac abnormalities should have antibiotics before dental or surgical treatment.

Chemotherapy Where an organism has been isolated from blood cultures, antibiotics should be given according to sensitivities. In the absence of an organism, a combination of amoxycillin and an aminoglycoside (e.g. gentamicin) covers the commonest organisms. Treatment should be for at least 4–6 weeks, the first 2 weeks being intravenous. Underlying abscesses should be sought and drained.

Peripheral arterial disease
Intermittent claudication
Aetiology
Atheromatous narrowing of the arteries to the legs.
Smoking.
Diabetes.

Symptoms Calf pain, usually unilateral, on walking and relieved by stopping. Typically the pain occurs after a known distance, e.g. 'I walk for 150 yards and have to stop for a few minutes and can then walk a further 150 yards.'

Signs

Diminished or absent femoral pulses, often with superimposed bruit.

The foot pulses (dorsalis pedis and posterior tibial pulses) may be difficult to feel or impalpable on the affected side.

Management Remove risk factors (stop smoking, lose weight, treat diabetes if present).

Endarterectomy to remove atheromatous plaque or femoral artery bypass surgery is the only available cure.

Acute arterial obstruction

Aetiology Tight atheromatous thrombosis or arterial embolism, most commonly in the femoral artery.

Symptoms

Severe pain and numbness in affected limb.

Shock with pallor and cold sweat.

Signs Remember the five Ps of an ischaemic limb:

Perishing cold

Pulseless

Pallor

Pain

Paraesthesia

Other signs are: tachycardia and hypotension.

Management Urgent surgical removal of embolus or arterial endarterectomy or bypass.

Raynaud's phenomenon

Intermittent arterial spasm affecting fingers and toes, precipitated by cold (weather and water).

Aetiology

No known cause (90%).

Connective tissue disease (rheumatoid arthritis, SLE).

Cold agglutinins (circulating immunoglobulins which precipitate in the cold).

Beta-blockade.

Cervical rib (arterial compression).

Symptoms Intermittent symmetrical pain and coldness of digits with typical colour changes:

- white – from arterial spasm;
- blue – as blood becomes anoxic;
- red – as spasm resolves and blood supply returns.

Management

Treat underlying cause if present (SLE, cervical ribs, beta-blocking drugs).

Avoid cold water.

Keep digits warm in cold weather.

Aortic abdominal aneurysm

Aetiology Atheromatous damage to aortic wall.

Symptoms Often asymptomatic and detected on routine abdominal examination or seen on abdominal X-ray.

Signs

Pulsatile abdominal aorta.

Bruits may be heard from nearby atheromatous arteries.

Complications Spontaneous rupture carries 80% mortality.

Management Consider surgical replacement with aortic graft if aneurysm more than 6 cm diameter – confirm with X-ray or CT scan – to prevent possible rupture.

Peripheral vein disease
Varicose veins of the legs

Varicose (dilated) veins are found in four main sites: the anal canal (haemorrhoids), the gastro-oesophageal junction in portal hypertension, around the testes (varicocoele) and in the legs. The commonest site is the legs.

Aetiology Incompetent valves between superficial and deep veins.

Symptoms

Large dilated veins are unsightly.

Ankle oedema.

Pain in legs on standing.

Signs Large superficial veins and massive varicosities at sites of incompetent valves (e.g. 'saphena varix' at the sapheno-femoral junction).

Complications
Most are small and uncomplicated.

Varicose (venous stagnation) ulcer over medial malleolus.

Management
Injection of varicose vein with sclerosing agent.

Ligation of deep perforating veins and stripping of unsightly superficial veins.

Deep venous thrombosis of leg

Aetiology
Previous trauma to leg (e.g. fractured tibia).

Prolonged stasis — bed rest after illness or surgery, long car or plane journey, rarely pressure on iliac veins or inferior vena cava (IVC) from abdominal tumour.

Malignancy at distant sites (e.g. pancreas, bronchus) predisposes to venous thrombosis.

Coagulation defects (e.g. antithrombin III deficiency).

Oral contraceptive pill.

Symptoms Swelling and pain in calf.

Signs Red, hot, swollen calf (compare diameter with other leg).

Investigations Doppler ultrasound may reveal clots, particularly in large veins. Otherwise the diagnosis should be confirmed by venography. The differential diagnosis is usually from a rupture of a Baker's cyst (synovial lined cyst behind the knee, connecting with the knee joint).

Complications Pulmonary embolism.

Management Anticoagulation for 6–8 weeks if otherwise uncomplicated.

Pulmonary embolism

Aetiology Deep venous thrombosis.

Symptoms

Haemoptysis.

Pleuritic chest pain.

Episodic breathlessness (from small recurrent emboli).

Acute breathlessness and marked anxiety (large embolus).

Circulatory collapse (massive embolus).

Signs

Anxiety.

Dyspnoea and tachypnoea.

Cyanosis.

Pleural rub.

Shock with coldness, clammy skin, tachycardia and hypotension, raised JVP, loud pulmonary second heart sound.

Investigations

CXR for elevation of hemidiaphragm on affected side, areas of infarction and heart size.

ECG for evidence of right heart strain (right axis deviation, tall R wave and T wave inversion in leads over right ventricle, right bundle branch block, rarely S_1, Q_3, T_3 pattern) (p. 307).

Blood gases for Pa_{O_2}.

Ventilation/perfusion scan (p. 280) for mismatched defects (perfusion defect with normal ventilation).

Management

Prevent with subcutaneous heparin prior to surgery and for prolonged bed rest.

Small and medium-size emboli Anticoagulation with IV heparin followed by warfarin for 3 months.

Oxygen.

Analgesia.

Large emboli and shock Surgical removal of clot from pulmonary arteries (see Emergencies, p. 230)

GASTROINTESTINAL DISEASES

The commonest presenting features are indigestion (see History, p. 15), diarrhoea (p. 27), constipation (p. 27) and abdominal pain (pp. 23–4)

Hiatus hernia and gastro-oesophageal reflux

Aetiology Weakness of diaphragmatic sphincter allows lower oesophagus and cardia of stomach to rise into thorax. Gastro-oesophageal reflux may occur in the presence or absence of a hiatus hernia, and is aggravated by smoking or alcohol.

Symptoms

Retrosternal burning pain, usually episodic.

'Acid' regurgitation into throat.

Worse on lying flat or bending.

Relieved by milk and antacids.

Flatulence, which may also give relief.

Signs None.

Investigations Only if persistent and symptoms severe or if associated with dysphagia (exclude benign or malignant stricture; p. 284) or weight loss (exclude oesophageal or gastric carcinoma; p. 285).

Barium swallow (p. 280) will reveal the hernia and the presence of gastric acid reflux.

Endoscopy will reveal the severity of oesophagitis.

Management

Reduce weight and stop smoking.

Avoid clothes which constrict and increase intra-abdominal pressure.

Raise head of the bed.

Avoid foods which induce symptoms, if known.

Antacids for symptoms.

Metoclopramide (promotes gastric emptying) and H_2-receptor antagonists if severe.

Surgery for hiatus hernia is very rarely indicated in the absence of stricture formation, as it is a major procedure and the results are uncertain.

Duodenal ulceration

Aetiology

Gastric acid hypersecretion (rarely gastrin-secreting tumour in Zollinger—Ellison syndrome).

Helicobacter pylori infection (predominantly gastric antral mucosa).

Symptoms

Periodic epigastric pain, radiating through to back if pancreas is inflamed by the ulcer (i.e. posterior duodenal ulcers).

Pain often wakes patient at 1–3 a.m.

Relieved by food, milk and antacids.

Signs Epigastric tenderness on palpation.

Investigations

Barium meal.

Fibreoptic endoscopy with biopsy of gastric antrum for *H. pylori*.

Complications

Haematemesis — acute bleed from ruptured vessel at ulcer base.

Perforation releasing gastric contents into abdominal cavity (peritonitis with generalized tenderness and board-like abdominal rigidity).

Pyloric stricture from recurrent inflammation followed by healing by fibrous tissue causes persistent vomiting.

Management

Stop smoking.

Avoid foods which give pain (e.g. usually onions, spices, bananas, alcoholic spirits).

Antacids for pain (e.g. magnesium trisilicate, aluminium hydroxide).

Gel antacids (e.g. Asilone gel, Mucaine), which coat the ulcer much as gastric mucus.

H_2 receptor blockers (e.g. cimetidine, ranitidine).

Hydrogen ion (H^+) (proton pump) blockers (e.g. omeprazole).

Helicobacter pylori infection can be suppressed with bismuth and antibiotics (ampicillin or tetracycline with metronidazole).

Surgery for:

- severe persistent symptoms destroying normal living;
- haematemesis if severe or repeated;
- perforation;
- pyloric stricture.

Gastric ulceration (benign or malignant ulcers)

Aetiology

Chronic gastric ulceration

Cigarette smoking.

Decreased protective gastric mucus bicarbonate secretion or mucosal blood flow.

Acute superficial

Aspirin and non-steroidal anti-inflammatory agents.

Prednisolone.

Stress (Cushing's ulcer).

Burns (Curling's ulcer).

Symptoms As duodenal ulcer but:

- vomiting more common — suggests carcinoma;
- weight loss more common — suggests carcinoma;
- dysphagia — suggests carcinoma of gastric cardia.

Investigations

Blood for anaemia — suggests carcinoma.

Barium meal (p. 280) to define ulcer.

Fibreoptic gastroscopy and tissue biopsy to distinguish benign from malignant ulcers.

Management

Benign gastric ulcers — as for duodenal ulcers.

Surgery for persistent severe symptoms, carcinoma, bleeding.

Haematemesis (see Emergencies, p. 238).

Irritable bowel disease (spastic colon)

Aetiology Possibly altered and irregular smooth muscle contraction in large intestinal wall.

Symptoms

Recurrent left or right iliac fossa pain relieved by defaecation.

Constipation or diarrhoea.

Signs

Tenderness over sites of pain.

Palpable loaded colon in left iliac fossa (LIF).

Investigations (to exclude serious underlying diseases)

Blood count for anaemia, ESR and CRP.

Stools for occult ('invisible') bleeding and culture.

Sigmoidoscopy to exclude ulcerative colitis.

Barium enema if faecal occult blood (FOB) positive, symptoms severe, alternate constipation and diarrhoea or weight loss, to exclude colonic carcinoma: will also reveal diverticular disease.

Management

High-fibre diet to 'retrain' bowel (bran, Fybogel).

Smooth muscle relaxants, e.g. mebeverine (Colofac).

NB: Always consider the possibility of colitis (Crohn's or ulcerative) and colonic carcinoma.

Acute appendicitis

Aetiology Obstruction to appendix lumen by phlebolith.

Symptoms

Abdominal pain – beginning around umbilicus and moving to right iliac fossa.

Nausea and vomiting.

Signs

Fever.

Abdominal tenderness and rebound over right lower abdomen (McBurney's point – halfway between umbilicus and right anterior iliac spine).

Complications

Rupture – peritonitis.

Appendix abscess if not removed but partially resolved with antibiotics.

Management Surgical removal.

Common anal disorders
Haemorrhoids

Varices of superior haemorrhoidal veins.

Symptoms and signs

Rectal bleeding (first degree – visible only on proctoscopy).

Prolapse on defaecation (second degree).

Persistent prolapse (third degree).

Rectal pain (severe) if the piles thrombose.

Mucous secretion and anal irritation.

Management

Anaesthetic creams and suppositories.

Increase dietary fibre to avoid constipation.

Sclerosing injections (first and second degree).

Haemorrhoidectomy (third degree).

Anal fissure

A tear at the anorectal margin.

Symptoms and signs

Acute severe anal pain.

Rectal bleeding.

Rectal examination is excruciatingly painful and anal sphincter in spasm; therefore anaesthetize anorectum first.

Fissure may be visible on proctoscopy.

Management

Local anaesthetics will help symptoms and prevent constipation.

Increase dietary fibre.

Anal stretch for persistent fissures.

Excision for chronic fissures if anal stretch ineffective.

Inflammatory bowel disease (ulcerative colitis (UC) and Crohn's)

Aetiology Unknown.

Symptoms

Abdominal pain.

Weight loss.

Altered bowel habit.

Passage of blood and mucus on defaecation.

Signs

Abdominal tenderness.

May be associated arthritis, skin rash (including erythema nodosum), uveitis, hepatitis.

Investigation

Blood for full blood count, ESR, CRP, liver function.

Sigmoidoscopy — rectum 'always' abnormal in UC, may be spared in Crohn's. Biopsy reveals superficial inflammation in UC, granulomas and deeper inflammation in Crohn's.

Barium enema (p. 288).

Small bowel follow-through if ileal Crohn's suspected.

Management

UC

Aminosalicylates (sulphasalazine, mesalazine).

Steroids topically in the form of suppositories or enemas.

Azathioprine may help maintain remission.

Crohn's

Colonic — as for UC.

Small bowel — exclusion diet and metronidazole may help.

Severe acute attacks

Systemic steroids.

Parenteral nutrition (with vitamin and potassium supplements).

Surgery if no improvement (or long-standing disease unresponsive to treatment-increased risk of colorectal carcinoma).

Malabsorption

Aetiology Coeliac disease (gluten-sensitive enteropathy) is commonest cause.

Rarer causes: tropical sprue, Whipple's disease, small bowel lymphoma, pancreatic disease.

Symptoms

Weight loss.

Abdominal discomfort.

Diarrhoea.

Signs

Of nutritional deficiencies — thin, oedema, glossitis, neuropathy.

Clubbing.

Diagnosis Coeliac disease: jejunal biopsy whilst on gluten diet (villous atrophy) and after introduction of gluten-free diet (normal).

Management If diagnosis is confirmed, continue gluten-free diet (gluten found in wheat, rye, barley but not rice, maize, soya).

THE LIVER, GALL BLADDER AND PANCREAS

Jaundice (see also p. 256)

Yellow discoloration of the sclera (whites of the eyes) and, if severe, the skin.

Working classification

Pre-hepatic (unrelated to liver disease)

Haemolytic anaemias.

Jaundice mild ('yellow tinge to eyes').

Hepatic

Acute viral hepatitis* (hepatitis A, B, C; glandular fever).

Drug toxicity (paracetamol overdose).

Metastatic malignant deposits.*

Jaundice mild to moderate.

Post-hepatic (obstructive jaundice)

Gallstone obstruction to bile duct.*

Carcinoma of pancreatic head* or biliary tract (cholangio-carcinoma).

* Denotes most common.

Jaundice marked. Pale (putty-coloured) stools, dark urine.
NB: Some drugs (e.g. chlorpromazine) cause an obstructive jaundice.

Liver failure

See Emergencies, p. 239.

Acute cholecystitis

Aetiology Usually associated with gallstones.

Symptoms

Right subcostal abdominal pain radiating round chest to angle of right scapula.

Fever and rigors.

Signs Acute tenderness over gall bladder.

Investigations Ultrasound of gall bladder for stones. Isotope scan may show increased uptake in gall bladder.

Management

Bed rest.

Analgesics (pethidine).

Antibiotics (cefotaxime: one-third of gall bladder coliforms are resistant to amoxycillin and trimethoprim).

Remove gall bladder in 2–3 weeks after acute inflammation settled.

(Some surgeons remove gall bladder during acute attack.)

Complications

Recurrence often associated with gallstones.

Chronic abscess (empyema of gall bladder).

Perforation — peritonitis.

NB: Gallstones are usually symptom-free but may cause:

• acute cholecystitis;

• chronic (recurrent) cholecystitis;

• obstructive jaundice;

• ascending cholangitis (Charcot's triad of fever, jaundice, right subcostal pain);

and are associated with pancreatitis and carcinoma of the gall bladder.

Acute pancreatitis

Aetiology

Usually unknown.

Alcohol, mumps, gallstone obstruction to pancreatic duct.

Symptoms Severe, often acute, generalized abdominal pain (patients hold themselves still as movement gives pain); pain radiates through centre of abdomen to back.

Signs

Tenderness with rebound on abdominal palpation.

Hypotension with sweating.

Cyanosis.

Rarely, bruising (chemical damage) in flanks or around the umbilicus.

Differential diagnosis

Acute cholecystitis if mild.

Perforated duodenal ulcer.

Dissection of aorta.

Myocardial infarction.

Mesenteric artery occlusion.

Investigations Markedly elevated serum amylase.

Ultrasound or CT scan may reveal a swollen pancreas.

Management

Analgesia with pethidine or phenazocine.

Gastric aspiration and intravenous fluid replacement.

Propantheline to block vagus and relax sphincter.

Monitor for and treat hyperglycaemia and hypocalcaemia.

Carcinoma of pancreas

Head (75%), body and tail (25%).

Symptoms and signs

Anorexia and weight loss.

Epigastric pain (indicative of duodenal or gastric ulceration) radiates through to back.

Jaundice with pale (putty) stools and dark urine (obstructive jaundice) if tumour in pancreatic head or in ampulla of Vater.

Investigations Abdominal ultrasound or CT may demonstrate tumour and enlarged bile ducts if obstructed.

Management Surgical removal of tumour if resectable at time of clinical presentation (ampullary and carcinoma of head present early, with obstructive jaundice).

Endoscopic retrograde cholangiopancreatography (ERCP) confirms the diagnosis and allows passage of a tube (stent) through an obstruction.

Islet cell tumour (insulinoma)
> Tumour of islet cells secretes excess insulin, causing recurrent hypoglycaemia.

Gastrinoma (from pancreas or stomach wall)
> Secretes excess gastrin, stimulating H^+ secretion and causing recurrent multiple duodenal and jejunal ulceration (Zollinger−Ellison syndrome).

UROGENITAL SYSTEM

Urinary tract infection
> There are two main clinical syndromes: acute cystitis and acute pyelonephritis.

Acute cystitis
> Urethral pain on micturition plus frequency (day and night).
> ### Aetiology
> > Bacterial infection (*Escherichia coli* in 95%).
> > Trauma — 'honeymoon cystitis'.
> ### Investigations
> > Stick testing of urine shows protein and usually blood.
> > MSU shows WBC and more than 100 000 organisms/ml.
> > Culture MSU for bacteria.
> > *NB*: Investigate further with ultrasound and/or intravenous urography for recurrent attacks. If uncommon organism grown (e.g. *Proteus*, *Klebsiella*, *Pseudomonas*) and if haematuria occurs, consider proceeding to cystoscopy to exclude:
> > - anatomical abnormality;
> > - stones;
> > - tumours.
> ### Management
> > Oral fluids.
> > Antibiotics (e.g. Augmentin or trimethoprim, depending upon bacterial sensitivity).
> > Surgery to remove stones or tumours.

Acute pyelonephritis
> Dysuria (pain on micturition), frequency, fever with rigors,

vomiting and loin tenderness over inflamed kidney (just below rib margin posteriorly).

Investigations As for acute cystitis but investigate fully after first attack.

Management Antibiotics often given IV as nausea is common, and to ensure rapid and effective blood levels.

Otherwise, manage as for acute cystitis.

Acute renal failure
See Emergencies, p. 240.

Nephrotic syndrome
A triad of:
- severe proteinuria (usually greater than 5 g/24 hours);
- hypoalbuminaemia;
- oedema of ankles and sometimes hands and face (periorbital).

NB: Hypercholesterolaemia is common.

Aetiology
Minimal-change glomerulonephritis (80% in children, 20% in adults).

Other forms of glomerulonephritis.

Systemic diseases, e.g. diabetes; SLE; multiple myelomatosis; drugs (e.g. gold, penicillamine); renal vein thrombosis.

Symptoms and signs Urine may be frothy (protein increases surface tension). Ankle oedema is usually the first sign. Fluid may also collect in the abdomen (ascites causing distension), in the lungs (pleural effusions causing breathlessness) and around eyes (which appear puffy).

Hypercoagulability occurs due to combination of hypovolaemia and clotting factor abnormalities.

Investigation
Serum albumin and 24-hour urine protein loss.

Renal function serum electrolytes, urea and creatinine, and glomerular filtration rate (GFR).

Investigate cause, including renal biopsy for histology.

Treatment
Treat underlying cause.

Diuretics.

Consider aspirin or anticoagulants to prevent venous thrombosis.

Prostatic hypertrophy

A common disorder of elderly men.

Symptoms

Early Difficulty starting micturition (hesitancy), narrow weak urinary stream, terminal dribbling following micturition.

Late Acute urinary retention with total anuria.

Signs

Tender palpable enlarged bladder in suprapubic region.

Rectal examination reveals enlarged prostate.

Investigations

Blood for elevated urea and creatinine concentration.

Ultrasound to show enlarged and dilated renal collecting systems (hydronephrosis) and prostate size.

NB: If retention continues (i.e. for days or weeks), symptoms and signs of renal failure ensue (p. 240).

Management

Early Transurethral resection of prostate (TURP).

Late Release urethral obstruction by urethral catheterization. TURP when renal function returned to normal.

Kidney and bladder stones

Aetiology

Urinary stasis (secondary to anatomical abnormality or partial outflow obstruction).

High solute concentration (e.g. dehydration, urate stones in gout).

Infection causing scarring of renal tissue.

Types

Calcium phosphate.

Calcium oxalate.

Urate.

Cystine.

Clinical features

Renal colic – pain from loin to groin and patient rolls in agony.

Suprapubic pain with bladder stones.

Cystitis and frequency.

Haematuria.

Investigations

MSU for infection.

Screen urine for cystine.

24-hour urine for calcium, phosphate, oxalate.

Blood for calcium, phosphate and uric acid.

Abdominal X-ray to visualize stone (90% radio-opaque).

Ultrasound or intravenous urography (IVU) to exclude urinary tract obstruction (pp. 286–90).

Management

Ureteric stones often pass spontaneously – catch stone for analysis (by sieving urine).

Pethidine for renal and ureteric colic.

Surgical removal by

Cystoscopy and ureteric exploration (for ureteric stones).

Ultrasonic disintegration (lithotripsy).

Cystotomy or nephro lithotomy.

Renal tract tumours

Kidney

Benign

Adenoma.

Haemangioma.

Papilloma of renal pelvis.

Malignant

Nephroblastoma (Wilm's tumour of children).

Hypernephroma* (adenocarcinoma).

Transitional cell carcinoma.

Squamous cell carcinoma.

Hypernephroma presents

- Usually with painless haematuria;
- as mass in loin;
- as pyrexia of unknown origin;
- with malignant spread ('cannon ball' metastases in lungs).

Bladder

Benign Papilloma.

Malignant

Transitional cell carcinoma.*

Squamous cell carcinoma.*

Adenocarcinoma.

* Denotes most frequent.

Sarcoma.
Clinical presentation
Usually painless haematuria.
Sometimes infection with dysuria.
Secondary spread to lungs.

Prostate
Benign Hypertrophy* (benign prostatic hypertrophy, BPH; see p. 186).
Malignant Adenocarcinoma.*
Clinical features of adenocarcinoma
As for benign hypertrophy (p. 186).
Haematuria.
Bony pain from secondary deposits (white and sclerotic on X-ray), usually in pelvis and vertebrae.
Small hard nodule on rectal examination.
NB: Confirm with elevated serum acid phosphatase and prostate specific antigen, and with prostatic biopsy per rectum.

Vaginal prolapse
Prolapse of vagina downward, secondary to weakening from age or following surgery, to the pelvic floor muscles.
Clinical features
Urinary incontinence on coughing or lifting, i.e. by increasing intra-abdominal pressure — a very common symptom in elderly women.
Prolapse, if severe, is palpable at vaginal orifice.
Vaginal prolapse visible on coughing during speculum examination.
Management
Hold prolapse with ring pessary inserted against vaginal vault.
Surgical repair.

Common gynaecological tumours
Fibroids
Benign myometrial tumours of uterus.
Clinical features
Menorrhagia (heavy periods containing blood clots).
Exhaustion from iron-deficiency anaemia.

Palpable suprapubically or on vaginal palpation.
Management of symptomatic fibroids
Surgical removal of tumour.

Hysterectomy if childbirth no longer contemplated.

Endometrial carcinoma
Usually post-menopausal in 50–60-year age group.
Clinical features
Post-menopausal vaginal bleeding.

Palpable tumour if presents late.

Diagnosis Carcinoma cells on endometrial biopsy or curettage (dilatation of cervix with endometrial curettage (D&C)).
Clinical staging
  0 Carcinoma *in situ* (in endometrial wall only: 90%).

   I Carcinoma confined to body of uterus: 70–90% (5-year survival).

  II Carcinoma of body and spread to cervix.

 III Extension into pelvis.

 IV Widespread extension to bladder or rectal mucosa and beyond.

Cervical carcinoma
Commonest in 40–55-year age group.
Clinical features
Irregular and intermenstrual bleeding.

Post-menopausal bleeding.

Diagnosis By cervical smear or biopsy.
Clinical staging
  0 Carcinoma *in situ*.

   I Carcinoma confined to cervix.

  II Invasion beyond cervix but not to pelvic wall.

 III Invasion to involve other pelvic tissues.

 IV Spread beyond pelvis.
Management
Carcinoma in situ Local excision by cone biopsy or laser.

Invasive Surgery or radiotherapy, alone or in combination.

Ovarian carcinoma
Commonest in 50–60-year age group.

Clinical features

Lower abdominal discomfort.

Abdominal swelling — suprapubic.

Anaemia and ascites are late features.

Lower abdominal mass palpable suprapubically or on vaginal examination.

Staging

I   Tumour limited to ovaries.

II   Extension from ovaries to surrounding pelvis.

III   Intraperitoneal or retroperitoneal spread.

IV   Distant extrapelvic metastases.

Management

Total hysterectomy with bilateral salpingo-oöphorectomy.

Radiotherapy.

NEUROLOGICAL DISEASE

Headache

The commonest presenting neurological symptom. There are rarely any helpful neurological signs. Stress is a commonly considered 'cause' though often impossible to substantiate. Common causes include sinusitis, dental infection and migraine.

Migraine

Typical features

Aura, e.g. bright lights, nausea, abdominal pain (cerebral vasoconstriction).

Severe unilateral headache or facial pain (cerebral vasodilatation).

Nausea and vomiting.

Rarely, transient hemianopia, hemiplegia, hemianaesthesia.

Investigation

Diagnosis usually made on history.

CT scan if persistent neurological signs or migraine always on same side.

Management

Stop the contraceptive pill.

Metoclopramide for nausea.

Aspirin or paracetamol for pain.

Prophylaxis — prevent cerebral vasoconstriction — propranolol, clonidine or pizotifen.

Trigeminal neuralgia
Typical features
Over-50s.

Agonizing lancing pain along fifth nerve distribution.

Periodic (e.g. for 4 weeks once or twice per year).

Absence of abnormal neurological signs between attacks.
Management
Carbamazepine is often effective.

Destruction of the Gasserian ganglion (e.g. by alcohol injection) may be required in severe cases.

Temporal arteritis
Typical features
Over-50s; intracranial vessels may be involved.

Scalp tenderness on combing and brushing.

Pain worse on pressure over temporal arteries

ESR usually over 70 mm/hour.

Temporal artery biopsy shows granulomatous arteritis in 60–80%.

Management Steroid urgently to prevent ophthalmic artery occlusion.

Raised intracranial pressure (from hypertension, tumours)
Typical features
Headache on waking.

Nausea and vomiting.

Papilloedema.

NB: Seek urgent expert advice to identify and treat underlying cause.

Cerebrovascular disease (cerebrovascular accidents (CVAs), strokes)
Classification
Intracerebral

Haemorrhage* 20%.

* Denotes most common.

Thrombosis or infarction* 80%.

Transient ischaemic attacks* (carotid or vertebral distribution).

Extracerebral

Extradural haemorrhage.

Subdural haemorrhage — often follows minor trauma in the elderly and causes fluctuating headache, drowsiness and confusion.

Subarachnoid haemorrhage.*

Intracerebral thrombosis and haemorrhage

Aetiology Hypertension, hyperlipidaemia, diabetes mellitus, contraceptive pill, smoking, obesity.

Clinical features

Acute onset of contralateral hemiplegia (internal capsule supplied by striate branches of middle cerebral artery — commonest site of occlusion).

Acute onset of hemianaesthesia.

Acute onset of homonymous, hemianopia (optic radiation damaged at isthmus below internal capsule).

Expressive dysphasia (if motor speech area damaged).

NB: Disability depends upon extent of bleed or ischaemia, e.g. small lesion — weakness or clumsiness of hand; extensive lesion — complete paralysis of arm and leg, or death.

NB: Cerebral embolism much less common and usually in presence of atrial fibrillation — features may be identical.

Management

Care of unconscious patient if severe (nursing, nutrition, fluids, bladder, physiotherapy).

Regular turning to prevent bed sores if patient immobile.

Physiotherapy.

Speech therapy if dysphasic or dyarthric (p. 109).

Transient ischaemic attacks (mini-strokes)

Sudden focal neurological disorders which settle completely within 24 hours with full functional recovery and no persistently abnormal signs.

Aetiology Platelet emboli from carotid or cerebrobasilar arteries.

Symptoms

Carotid Amaurosis fugax (transient unilateral blindness as a result of ophthalmic artery embolism).

Cerebral Transient hemiplegia (internal capsule).

Brain stem Transient vertigo with nystagmus.

Drop attacks Sudden fall to the ground without loss of consciousness; usually in elderly and probably due to transient brain stem ischaemia.

Management

Treat hypertension, hyperlipidaemia.

Aspirin 75 mg daily.

Consider anticoagulation if atrial fibrillation or known source of emboli.

Subarachnoid haemorrhage

Aetiology
Acute bleed from ruptured congenital (Berry) aneurysm in circle of Willis (usually anterior communicating or middle cerebral posterior communicating arteries).

Clinical features

Acute severe pain in neck.

Photophobia.

Neck stiffness.

Collapse (irritable, confused).

Unconsciousness.

Death.

Investigations

Lumbar puncture (LP) reveals uniformly blood-stained cerebrospinal fluid (CSF) and xanthochromia (p. 267).

CT scan confirms diagnosis and extent of bleed (LP dangerous if raised intracranial pressure present).

Management

Care of unconscious patient.

Arteriography to define site of aneurysm with view to surgical clipping to prevent further bleed.

Nimodipine prevents cerebral ischaemia from vascular spasm.

Epilepsy

See causes of syncope p. 33 (with lists), and see also seizure classification below.

Aetiology

Electrical discharge in brain detected on encephatogram (EEG), which may be 'focal' or 'generalized'. Stimulation by TV, disco strobes, alcohol.

Usually idiopathic (no cause found).

Cerebral tumour, abscess or angioma.

Follows severe head injury.

Follows neurosurgery.

Clinical features of grand mal

Aura (e.g. impending doom, abdominal pain).

Coma and tonic phase — rigid, 30 seconds absent respiration with cyanosis.

Clonic — jerking of limbs, micturition, tongue biting.

Sleep — 1–3 hours

Acute management

Leave where fallen unless dangerous.

Roll into coma position on side.

Keep your fingers out of their mouth.

Wait and observe.

Rectal or IV diazepam for repeated frequent fits.

(Care — may require incubation and artificial ventilation if high dose required for sedation.)

NB: Jacksonian (focal) fits begin at one site, e.g. thumb, and may proceed to affect whole body.

Clinical features of temporal lobe

Hallucinations (*déjà vu*).

Visual disturbance (e.g. micropsia or macropsia — things look smaller or larger than they are).

Olfactory and gustatory auras.

Automatism — complex quasi-rational movement pattern.

May proceed to grand mal fits.

Clinical features of petit mal

Children and adolescents.

Moments of absence (daydreaming).

Akinetic seizures.

Myoclonic (sudden limb) jerks.

EEG with 'spike and wave' at three per second.

Management of epileptic attacks Phenytoin or carbamazepine for grand mal and temporal lobe or petit mal.

Sodium valproate may also be of benefit.

NB: Legal driving restrictions until epilepsy controlled.

Multiple sclerosis

Aetiology Demyelination of central nervous system (CNS) white matter of unknown cause.

Affects

Optic and ophthalmic nerves (II, III, IV, VI).

Brain stem.

Cerebellum and connections.

Dorsal (position and vibration sense) and lateral (pyramidal) tracts.

Clinical features

Transient and recurrent neurological defects

Retrobulbar neuritis with blurred vision.

Diplopia from third, fourth and sixth nerve palsy or brain stem demyelination.

Upper motor neurone unilateral weakness of limbs.

Sensory deficit in limbs — unilateral.

Disturbed micturition — precipitancy is common.

Cerebellar signs (from brain stem demyelination)

Nystagmus, dysarthria, intention tremor.

Diagnosis MRI scan for demyelination plaques (p. 293).

Management Physiotherapy and rehabilitation. Steroids reduce the duration of acute attacks.

Parkinson's disease

Aetiology Deficiency of dopamine in extrapyramidal system (caudate lobe, lentiform nucleus and thalamus). The normal balance between the neurotransmitters dopamine and acetylcholine is upset such that there is a relative excess of acetylcholine and lack of dopamine.

Parkinsonian symptoms may also be induced by the major tranquillizers such as phenothiazines (e.g. chlorpromazine) and butyrophenones (e.g. haloperidol).

Clinical features

Rigidity, tremor, bradykinesia (slow movement).

Flat affect and expressionless face.

Difficulty initiating movement (akinesia).

Rigid limbs — shuffling gait and arms do not swing with walking.

Speech slurred and monotonous.

Tremor — pill rolling, worse at rest.

Cogwheel rigidity of muscles — best felt on moving wrists.

Depression.

Management

Levodopa (as Sinemet or Madopar when combined with a dopa-decarboxylase inhibitor to prevent extracerebral effects).

Benzhexol (antimuscarinic).

Selegiline (monoamine oxidase inhibitor (MAOI)).

Bromocriptine (dopamine agonist).

Motor neurone disease

Aetiology Progressive degeneration of anterior horn cells of spinal cord, cells of lower cranial motor nuclei or neurones of motor cortex with secondary degeneration of pyramidal tracts. Cause unknown.

Clinical features Muscle weakness and fasciculation in the absence of sensory signs. Three classical patterns are recognized:

• lower motor neurone weakness of hands, progressing to involve upper and lower limbs ('progressive muscular atrophy');

• bulbar palsy;

• upper motor neurone weakness of limbs ('amyotrophic lateral sclerosis').

Progressive weakness usually leads to death from aspiration pneumonia or respiratory failure.

Myasthenia gravis

Aetiology Myasthenia gravis is an autoimmune disorder in which there are antibodies against the acetylcholine receptor. A thymoma is present in 10% of patients.

Clinical features Painless muscle weakness, worse towards the end of the day, and usually most marked in the face and eyes (may present with diplopia). Proximal muscles are affected more than distal. There is no wasting and tendon reflexes are normal.

Diagnosis Edrophonium (Tensilon, anticholinesterase — prolongs action of acetylcholine by inhibiting its breakdown) 10 mg IV (with cardiac monitor in case of bradycardia) produces a rapid but transient (up to 5 minutes) improvement in muscle weakness. Acetylcholine receptor antibodies are present in over 90% of patients.

Management Symptomatic treatment with oral long-acting cholinesterases (e.g. neostigmine, pyridostigmine). Thymectomy (even in the absence of thymoma) and immunosuppression (steroids with or without azathioprine) are of value in inducing remission or reducing disease progression.

Acute myasthenia gravis (myasthenic crisis)

Crisis usually occurs in patients with known myasthenia who are acutely unwell (e.g. influenza) or are given neuromuscular blocking agents as antibiotics (gentamicin) or anaesthetics (suxamethonium).

Management

Call for the cardiac arrest team or an anaesthetist urgently.

Edrophonium (Tensilon) 2 mg IV stat, repeating up to 8 mg with improvement.

NB: If edrophonium gives no response, this suggests that the myasthenic patient has been given excess anticholinesterase (pyridostigmine or neostigmine) – the even rarer cholinergic crisis.

Management of cholinergic crisis

Call for the cardiac arrest team.

Intubate and ventilate if experienced – otherwise give atropine 1 mg IV and await anaesthetist.

Hereditary ataxias

Aetiology Usually autosomal dominant disorders with progressive degeneration of one or more of: cerebellum, long ascending tracts in the spinal cord, optic nerves.

Clinical features Depend on particular disorder. In Friedreich's ataxia, cerebellar ataxia develops in teens, together with long tract signs (pyramidal and dorsal column) and optic atrophy. Cardiomyopathy causes arrhythmias and heart failure, the commonest cause of death.

Depression

Mild downswings of mood are usual. Severe mood swings are abnormal.

Clinical features

Sadness.

Feelings of uselessness and guilt.

Weepy spontaneously.

Difficulty sleeping and early waking.

Agitation or apathy.

Suicidal feelings — seek expert advice.

Management

Strong personal support — friend or doctor.

Tricyclic antidepressant agents (amitriptyline, mianserin, dothiepin).

MAOI (e.g. paroxetine).

Serotonin uptake inhibitors (e.g. paroxetine).

Anxiety

Normal with everyday stress. If it interferes with everyday life = anxiety.

Clinical features

Irrational worry.

Sweating, palpitation, tremor (adrenergic).

Phobias (agora (market place) — going out; claustro (cloister) — staying in).

Management

Psychological support.

Benzodiazepines for short-term relief of severe anxiety only.

CONNECTIVE TISSUE AND JOINT DISEASE

Osteoarthritis

Degenerative joint disease primarily of weight-bearing joints.

Pre-disposing factors

Age.

Obesity.

Trauma — jogging spines, sportsmen's knees.

Clinical features

Asymmetrical distribution.

Weight-bearing joints — spine, hip, knee; although any joint may be involved.

Pain on movement.

Deformity from bone overgrowth at articular margins.

Effusion with damaged joints.

Investigations X-ray shows loss of joint space (i.e. loss of cartilage), osteophytes at joint margins, bone cysts and sclerosis at articular surfaces.

Management

Weight and trauma reduction.

Analgesia with aspirin, paracetamol, non-steroidal anti-inflammatory drugs.

Surgical replacement for severe pain and/or deformity.

NB: Hallux valgus — marked osteoarthritic (OA) deformity of metatarsophalangeal joint of the big toe.

Rheumatoid arthritis

A generalized connective tissue disorder — joint disease is the prominent feature.

Clinical features

General — fever and intermittent or chronic ill health.

Joint disease — symmetrical involvement of wrists, fingers and other synovial joints (e.g. knees, elbows) with stiffness and pain on movement, and fixed deformity (e.g. ulnar deviation of wrist and fingers) if chronic.

Periarticular — soft tissue swelling and inflammation, tenosynovitis (e.g. Achilles tendinitis).

Skin — rash, subcutaneous nodules at elbow.

Lung — infiltration causing restrictive lung disease (nodules on X-ray).

Pericarditis.

Vasculitis — splinter haemorrhages at nailbed.

Neuropathy — peripheral, usually sensory.

Reticuloendothelial system — spleen and lymph node enlargement.

Eyes — keratoconjunctivitis sicca.

Sjögren's syndrome is the combination of rheumatoid arthritis with dry eyes and dry mouth (xerostomia) due to lacrimal and salivary gland infiltration.

Investigations

Normochromic, normocytic anaemia.

Raised ESR and CRP.

Positive rheumatoid factor (circulating immunoglobulin M (IgM) against patient's own IgG) in 80% of cases. (*NB*: In seronegative arthritis, such as psoriatic arthritis, ankylosing spondylitis and Reiter's disease, the rheumatoid factor is absent.)

Management Physiotherapy and non-steroidal anti-inflammatory drugs for joint stiffness and pain.

The disease process may be favourably influenced by a number of drugs including immunosuppressants (corticosteroids, azathioprine, cyclophosphamide), gold, chloroquine, penicillamine and sulphasalazine.

Gout

Inborn error of purine metabolism.

Clinical features

Swollen and red with excruciating joint pain, often in one first metatarsophalangeal joint though any other joint may be affected.

Fever.

Elevated blood uric acid.

Management

Rest painful joint.

Anti-inflammatory analgesia (e.g. indomethacin or naproxen).

Prophylaxis following repeated attacks with allopurinol (xanthine oxidase inhibitor which reduces the formation of uric acid from purines. Initiation of treatment may precipitate an attack of gout, so cover with an anti-inflammatory analgesic).

NB: Secondary gout from thiazide or loop diuretics, or myeloproliferative disorders on beginning therapy — massive cell destruction with purine release.

Systemic lupus erythematosus

Aetiology Unknown. Commoner in women aged 20−40. Certain drugs (e.g. hydralazine, procainamide) can induce an SLE-like syndrome.

Clinical features Extremely variable. Most are due to vasculitis (see below) affecting capillaries, arterioles and venules. Almost any organ can be involved, including skin (rashes, photosensitivity), joints (arthritis), kidneys (glomerulonephritis), nervous system (cranial or peripheral nerve lesions; CNS involvement leading to focal signs or psychiatric disturbance), cardiac (pericarditis, myocarditis), blood (anaemia, thrombocytopenia, leucopenia). The classical 'butterfly' rash on the face is often not present.

Diagnosis Antinuclear antibodies are positive in over 95% of patients. The majority of patients also have antibodies against double-stranded deoxyribonucleic acid (DNA) which are diagnostic. Anaemia, either associated with chronic disease (p. 244) or due to haemolysis (p. 245), is common. The ESR is raised in active disease. Biopsy of inflamed tissue characteristically shows vasculitis with deposition of immune (antigen–antibody) complexes and complement.

Management Immunosuppression with steroids, often in combination with cyclophosphamide or azathioprine. Chloroquine may be beneficial, particularly for skin lesions.

3

Systemic vasculitis

Aetiology Inflammation of small blood vessels occurs in a number of generalized inflammatory diseases, including microscopic polyarteritis and Wegener's granulomatosis. The cause is unknown, although flare-up of disease is often associated with infection.

Clinical features Many organs can be affected; common sites are skin, lungs, kidney, joints, eyes, nervous system. Clinical features include:

• malaise, fever, rashes, uveitis, arthritis;
• dyspnoea, cough, haemoptysis (from pulmonary haemorrhage);
• haematuria, renal failure (glomerulonephritis);
• psychiatric disturbance, epilepsy, strokes, peripheral neuropathy.

Diagnosis Over 90% of patients have positive anti-neutrophil cytoplasm antibodies.

Management Immunosuppression with steroids, usually in combination with cyclophosphamide or azathioprine.

Polymyositis

Aetiology Unknown. The finding of positive anti-nuclear antibodies or rheumatoid factor in some patients suggests an autoimmune disturbance. In patients over 50, particularly those with dermatomyositis (see below), an underlying malignancy may be present.

Clinical features Most commonly presents in women age 30–60 with muscle pain, tenderness and weakness, although any age or sex may be affected.

Proximal muscles are usually affected. Respiratory muscle involvement may endanger life, and oesophageal muscle involvement may cause dysphagia.

Raynaud's phenomenon, arthralgia and skin rashes are common.

Dermatomyositis is the combination of polymyositis and a typical rash with purple 'heliotrope' (a lilac-blue flower) like lesions around the eyes and over the small joints of the hands, often in association with telangiectasia (dilated capillaries and small arterioles) in the skin.

Diagnosis Muscle enzymes (creatine kinase, aldolase) are markedly elevated, reflecting active muscle destruction.

Electromyography (EMG) shows short-duration, low-amplitude, polyphasic action potentials (evidence of decreased active muscle), with spontaneous muscle fibre fibrillation (probably reflecting muscle irritability).

Muscle biopsy shows muscle fibre necrosis and inflammatory cell infiltration.

Management Immunosuppression with corticosteroids (together with azathioprine in resistant cases, or as a steroid sparing agent) is usually required for 1–3 years. Spontaneous remission may occur in the young, whereas the prognosis is worse in the elderly, in whom there may be an underlying malignancy. Physiotherapy is usually very helpful.

Scleroderma (systemic sclerosis)

Aetiology Unknown. A disease in which collagen fibres initially swell, and later become sclerotic, leading to fibrosis and atrophy of various structures, particularly the skin. Blood vessels show inflammation (vasculitis) and thickening.

Clinical features Predominantly affects middle-aged women. The skin (affected in 90% of cases) initially becomes smooth, waxy and tight, and later thin, atrophic and pigmented. The changes are maximal over the hands (fingers have the thin, shiny, elongated appearance of sclerodactyly), ankles and face.

Raynaud's phenomenon is common, and often precedes the other features.

Skin ulcers may develop.

Involvement of other systems may lead to dysphagia (oesophageal involvement), respiratory failure (pulmonary fibrosis or overspill of food into the lungs from oesophageal involvement) and renal involvement (usually arterial thickening with hypertension).

Arthralgia is common and skeletal muscle and cardiac muscle fibrosis may occur.

The CREST syndrome, a variant of systemic sclerosis, consists of:

Calcinosis (calcification of soft tissues, particularly in the fingers),

Raynaud's phenomcnon,

o**E**sophageal involvement,

Sclerodactyly and

Telangiectasia.

Morphoea is a localized skin form of scleroderma, with no evidence of systemic involvement. It is benign and rarely proceeds to systemic sclerosis.

Investigation The diagnosis is usually made on clinical grounds. Anti-nuclear antibodies are present in 80% of patients with systemic sclerosis.

Anti-centromere (the site at which the long and short arm of chromosomes join) antibodies are present in CREST syndrome.

Barium swallow may reveal oesophageal involvement, and hand X-rays may reveal soft tissue calcification.

Management No treatment has been shown to affect progression of the disease. Treatment is symptomatic — sleeping upright to prevent oesophageal reflux or overspill, anti-inflammatory agents for joints/muscles, heated gloves and avoiding cold for Raynaud's, anti-hypertensives.

Ankylosing spondylitis

Clinical features Young adult males — 96% HLA B27 (HLA stands for human leucocyte antigens, which together make up the major histocompatibility (MHC) class I and II antigens which enable cells to interact with lymphocytes in immune regulation. HLA B27 describes a type of class I antigen).

Articular Sacroileitis causing low back pain; may progress to involve lumbosacral region, thoracic and cervical spine, eventually causing spinal fusion.

Extra-articular

Uveitis.

Aortic regurgitation.

Ulcerative colitis.

Upper lobe pulmonary fibrosis.

Management

Analgesia.

Exercises and careful posture to prevent deformity.

Reiter's syndrome

Aetiology Usually occurs in young adult males (70% HLA B27) following gastrointestinal infection (*Shigella*, *Salmonella*, *Yersinia*, *Campylobacter*) or venereal infection.

Clinical features Triad of:
- arthritis (seronegative) — asymmetrical, polyarticular;
- urethritis;
- conjunctivitis.

Management Symptomatic with rest and analgesia whilst spontaneous resolution occurs — recurrence is common.

Marfan's syndrome

Aetiology Autosomal dominant connective tissue disorder affecting aortic media, eyes and skeleton.

Clinical features

Tall stature, long thin digits.

High arched palate.

Pectus excavatum (depressed sternum).

Dislocation of the lens of the eye.

Weakness of the aortic media predisposes to dilatation and dissection.

METABOLIC AND ENDOCRINE DISORDERS

Diabetes mellitus

The term diabetes means excessive urination (polyuria), which in diabetes mellitus is due to the osmotic diuretic effect of glucose. Diabetes insipidus refers to polyuria due to a deficiency of ADH or an inability of the kidneys to respond to ADH.

Half a million cases of diabetes mellitus are diagnosed in UK.

Presenting features

Glycosuria on routine testing.

Polyuria, polydipsia and weight loss.

Confusion or coma — usually keto-acidotic.

Aetiology Either autoimmune destruction of the pancreatic islet cells (usually young, insulin-dependent), pancreatic insufficiency from other causes (e.g. pancreatitis, carcinoma of the pancreas), resistance to insulin, drugs (e.g. steroids, thiazides) or other endocrine disorders (e.g. Cushing's syndrome).

Complications

Vascular — atheroma and coronary insufficiency; small-vessel ischaemia of feet.

Eye — background retinopathy — microaneurysms; exudates and haemorrhages; proliferative retinopathy — new vessel formation. (*NB*: New vessel formation — these may grow into the vitreous, causing retinal detachment, or rupture, causing sudden blindness.)

Kidney — pyelonephritis; glomerular and nodular sclerosis; chronic renal failure.

Nervous system — peripheral neuropathy affecting initially dorsal columns (position and vibration).

Intercurrent infection — may precipitate coma.

Management

Elderly, obese — diet (increase fibre, decrease refined carbohydrate (CHO)); oral hypoglycaemic agents.

Young, slim — diet; insulin.

Regular review — general health, hypoglycaemic and hyperglycaemic episodes from patient's home records.

Annual check for:

• visual acuity and fundal appearance;

- BP;
- insulin technique and injection sites;
- feet for infection and ulcers;
- diabetic control — home glucose monitoring, haemoglobin (Hb) A_1C.

Types of coma

Hypoglycaemia — anxiety, tachycardia, sweating, confusion — coma (see Emergencies p. 235).

Hyperglycaemic keto-acidosis (see Emergencies p. 235).

Hyperosmolar.

Myxoedema (hypothyroidism)

Clinical features

Slow onset.

Sensitivity to cold.

Weight gain.

Mental lethargy — dementia.

Coarse skin.

Hoarse voice.

Hair loss.

Investigations

Low T4.

High thyroid-stimulating hormone (TSH).

Thyroid autoantibodies are present in Hashimoto's (autoimmune) thyroiditis.

Management Thyroxine — start with $25-50\,\mu g$ daily and increase until TSH is suppressed into the normal range.

Thyrotoxicosis (hyperthyroidism)

Clinical features

Adrenergic — anxiety, tachycardia, sweating palms, fine finger tremor.

Eye signs — lid lag, exophthalmos, ophthalmic muscle weakness causing diplopia.

Thyroid gland enlargement (goitre) (Graves' disease: thyrotoxic symptoms with diffuse goitre and eye signs).

Investigations

T3 and T4 raised.

TSH zero (suppressed at the anterior pituitary).

Management There are three lines of therapy:
Anti-thyroid drugs (e.g. carbimazole).
Radio-iodine ablation of gland.
Surgery if medical treatment unsuccessful.

Cushing's syndrome

Aetiology The result of excess corticosteroids. The commonest cause is prolonged treatment with steroids. Other causes are an ACTH-secreting tumour of the pituitary gland (Cushing's disease), tumours of the adrenal gland (adenoma or carcinoma) or, rarely, ACTH-secreting tumours elsewhere (e.g. oat cell carcinoma of bronchus).

Clinical features
'Cushingoid appearance' — 'moon facies', truncal obesity ('buffalo hump'), purpura, striae, proximal muscle weakness and wasting.
Hypertension.
Osteoporosis.
Cataracts.
Carbohydrate intolerance (diabetes mellitus in about 10%).
Electrolyte disturbance (hypokalaemic alkalosis) due to mineralocorticoid effect.
Androgenic effects — acne, hirsutism, amenorrhoea.
Psychiatric disturbance.

Investigation Plasma cortisol is raised with loss of the normal diurnal variation (cortisol levels normally peak on waking).

ACTH levels are increased in pituitary-dependent Cushing's (or ACTH-secreting tumour) and suppressed in adrenal tumours.

Skull X-ray (enlarged pituitary fossa) and cranial CT are useful in identifying pituitary tumours. Abdominal CT helps identify adrenal hyperplasia or tumour.

Management Surgical removal of pituitary or adrenal tumours followed by cortisol replacement therapy where indicated.

Adrenal insufficiency
Rare — see p. 237.

3

Acromegaly

Aetiology Excess growth hormone causes gigantism in early life (before the epiphyses have closed) and acromegaly in adult life. The source is usually an eosinophilic pituitary adenoma.

Clinical features

Due to overgrowth of soft tissues, including the skin, tongue, viscera and bones.

Increased skull size (and hence hat size), prominent supra-orbital ridges and jaw.

Spade-shaped hands and feet — carpal tunnel syndrome (compression of the median nerve at the wrist) may occur.

Cardiomyopathy and hypertension (the main cause of increased mortality).

Glucose intolerance and diabetes due to anti-insulin effects of growth hormone.

Investigation

Plasma growth hormone level is raised and fails to show normal suppression during a glucose tolerance test (75 g of oral glucose).

Skull X-ray for enlargement of the pituitary fossa, and CT scan to detect the presence of an adenoma.

Visual fields by perimetry for bitemporal hemianopia.

Hand X-rays show tufting of the terminal phalanges and increased joint space (due to hypertrophy of cartilage).

Management

Surgical removal of tumour.

Yttrium-90 implants into the tumour or radiotherapy if surgery is contraindicated (e.g. in the elderly).

Bromocriptine reduces growth hormone levels, and is also useful for shrinking tumours prior to surgery.

Conn's syndrome (rare)

Aetiology Benign adenoma or hyperplasia of the zona glomerulosa (aldosterone-producing part) of the adrenal cortex.

Clinical features Secondary to sodium retention (hypertension, usually without oedema) and potassium loss (hypokalaemic muscle weakness).

Investigation

Hypokalaemic alkalosis with increased urinary potassium.

Serum aldosterone is increased and renin suppressed in a 7 a.m. sample from a rested recumbent patient.

Adrenal CT scan identifies adrenal tumours.

Management

Surgical resection of adrenal tumours.

Spironolactone antagonizes the effects of aldosterone.

Phaeochromocytoma

Rare, but important, treatable cause of hypertension.

Aetiology Usually benign tumour of adrenal medulla, but can occur in chromaffin tissue at other sites.

Clinical features

Due to excess catecholamine secretion (adrenaline — beta and some alpha adrenergic effects; noradrenaline — alpha effects).

Hypertension — may be paroxysmal and associated with tachycardia, sweating, anxiety and headache.

Investigation

Measure catecholamines in blood or urine (as the metabolite vanillylmandelic acid (VMA) in a 24-hour collection).

CT scan, initially of the abdomen, to localize the tumour (may be bilateral).

Management Remove tumour under full blockade of alpha (e.g. phentolamine) and beta (e.g. propranolol) adrenergic effects. Avoid beta-blockade alone in suspected phaeochromocytoma because of risk of hypertensive crisis from unopposed alpha effects.

Haemochromatosis

Aetiology Increased gastrointestinal iron absorption results in iron deposition in multiple organs. Autosomal recessive, but clinical features uncommon in females, who lose iron through menstruation.

Clinical features Are due to deposition of iron in liver (cirrhosis), pancreas (diabetes), heart (cardiomyopathy), pituitary (gonadal atrophy).

Pigmentation occurs as a result of both iron and melanin deposition in skin.

Investigation

Hb is normal but serum iron and ferritin are raised.

Liver function tests and glucose tolerance may be abnormal. Biopsy of most tissues (skin, marrow, liver) shows excess iron staining.

Diagnosis is usually confirmed by liver biopsy, which shows iron staining of liver cells with perilobular fibrosis.

Cirrhosis in advanced cases is associated with an increased risk of hepatocellular carcinoma.

Management Deplete the body of excess iron by regular venesection (500 ml once or twice weekly initially) until serum ferritin is within normal range. Specific treatment may be required for organ damage (e.g. insulin for diabetes).

Screen family members to detect asymptomatic disease.

Wilson's disease

Aetiology Autosomal recessive disorder of copper metabolism leading to excessive copper deposition in many organs, including liver, brain, kidneys and cornea.

Investigation Serum copper and the copper-carrying protein caeruloplasmin are low, and urinary copper increased.

Clinical features Cirrhosis (hepatic deposition), incoordination and involuntary movements (basal ganglia deposition), dementia (cerebral deposition) and renal tubular defects develop during adolescence or early adult life.

Kayser—Fleischer rings (a green-gold ring of copper deposition) around the cornea of the eye are pathognomic (only occur in, and therefore indicate the presence of, the disease).

Management Low dietary copper intake and penicillamine, which chelates copper and increases its urinary excretion. Screen family members.

Tetany

This results from *hypocalcaemia* (ionized calcium), usually following parathyroidectomy, and from *alkalosis* from hyperventilation (the hyperventilation or overbreathing syndrome in anxiety).

Clinical features Include paraesthesia (pins and needles with numbness) of the lips with carpopedal spasm (Trousseau's sign) and twitching of the angle of the mouth (Chvostek's sign) on percussing the seventh nerve as it leaves the stylomastoid foramen — nerves and muscles are more excitable in hypocalcaemia.

Emergency management

10 ml of 10% calcium gluconate IV.

Rebreathing from a paper bag if hyperventilation.

Toxic hypercalcaemia

Usually from calcium released from bone breakdown due to carcinomatous secondary deposits.

Clinical features Vomiting, polyuria, polydipsia preceding acute irritability, leading to confusion and coma.

Emergency management Reduce circulating calcium levels with:

- rehydration — normal saline 1 litre IV in half an hour;
- frusemide 80 mg IV;

Other slower methods include:

- bisphosphonates (e.g. pamidronate) IV (inhibit mobilization of calcium from skeleton);
- calcitonin IM.

SKIN DISORDERS

Eczema

Aetiology Usually occurs in atopic individuals (tendency to asthma, hay fever and eczema, often with a family history of these conditions).

Often exacerbated by diet or environmental factors (e.g. heat, drying of skin).

Clinical features

Redness, heat, swelling and irritation of affected area.

Usually affects flexural surfaces (elbow, wrist, ankle, knee, neck).

Vesicles may occur and rupture on scratching to cause weeping.

Management

Avoid perfumed soaps or 'bubble bath'.

Alleviate dryness of the skin with aqueous cream or emulsifying ointment.

Mild topical (i.e. locally applied) corticosteroid (e.g. 1% hydrocortisone).

Contact dermatitis

Aetiology Local eczematous reaction to an irritant in contact with skin.

Clinical features As for eczema but rash localized to specific area (e.g. skin in contact with a piece of jewellery, hands in contact with washing-up detergent).

Diagnosis Usually obvious from history. Patch testing (suspected allergen is placed in contact with skin, usually on back, and the site observed for a reaction) may confirm the diagnosis.

Management

Avoid known irritants.

Topical steroid to resolve acute episodes.

Psoriasis

Aetiology Unknown. Genetic factors are contributory.

Clinical features Well demarcated plaques with scaly surface predominantly over extensor surfaces (knees, elbows) and in the scalp.

Associated with arthritis and pitting of nails.

Management

Topical treatments

Coal tar and salicylate ointment.

Dithranol (discolours clothing).

Steroids, but avoid long-term use if possible.

Systemic

PUVA — oral psoralens and exposure to ultraviolet A (UVA) light.

Methotrexate.

Drug eruption

Aetiology Almost any drug can cause eruptions although the commonest include antibiotics (penicillins, sulphonamides), thiazides, allopurinol, ACE inhibitors.

Clinical features Any form of rash, including erythematous, maculopapular, urticarial or purpuric, may occur, and the pattern for any one drug is not always the same.

Certain associations are recognized (e.g. photosensitivity with phenothiazines, pigmentation with amiodarone, acne with steroids, maculopapular rash with ampicillin when given for infectious mononucleosis).

Management

Stop all drugs if possible.

Oral antihistamines.

Steroids may be required if severe.

Adrenaline may be life-saving in acute hypersensitivity reactions with shock or angioedema (p. 228).

Erythema nodosum

Aetiology Sarcoid, infections (streptococcal, TB, leprosy, psittacosis), inflammatory bowel disease, drugs (sulphonamides, oral contraceptives).

Clinical features Painful red nodules on the shins.

Investigation

Diagnosis is made on clinical appearance.

CXR to exclude sarcoid, infection.

Management

Rest.

Anti-inflammatory drugs (e.g. indomethacin).

BONE DISEASE

Osteoporosis

Reduced bone mass per unit of bone volume.

Aetiology Old age (particularly post-menopausal women — oestrogens prevent bone reabsorption), immobilization, corticosteroid therapy, Cushing's syndrome, hyperthyroidism, acromegaly, alcoholism.

Localized osteoporosis occurs around unused joints (e.g. in rheumatoid arthritis).

Clinical features Usually presents with skeletal pain secondary to fracture or vertebral collapse.

Investigation

Plain X-rays are of limited value except to exclude fracture.

Plasma calcium, phosphate and alkaline phosphatase are all normal (unless alkaline phosphatase raised following recent fracture).

Bone mass measurement confirms the diagnosis but is not widely available.

Underlying causes should be excluded.

Management

Treat any underlying cause.

Encourage mobility.

Oestrogen therapy is of value in post-menopausal women but carries the potential risk of endometrial carcinoma (use cyclical therapy). Ensure adequate dietary calcium. Established vertebral osteoporosis may respond to cyclical etidronate with calcium supplements.

Osteomalacia

Abnormal bone mineralization due to vitamin D deficiency. Cholecalciferol (from diet or synthesized in skin) is 25-hydroxylated in the liver, and then further hydroxylated to the active form (1,25-dihydroxycholecalciferol) in the kidney. 1,25-Dihydroxycholecalciferol increases intestinal absorption of calcium, and increases bone resorption and calcification.

Aetiology

Dietary deficiency/inadequate sunlight (particularly Asian women).

Malabsorption.

Renal disease (renal osteodystrophy is a combination of osteomalacia and hyperparathyroidism, which occurs as a secondary response).

Clinical features

Childhood Rickets — bone deformity (bow legs), inadequate growth.

Adults Bone pain, fractures; proximal myopathy.

Investigation

Low or normal plasma calcium, low plasma phosphate.

Increased alkaline phosphatase.

X-rays — defective mineralization, Looser's zones (p. 294).

Bone biopsy confirms the abnormal bone mineralization.

Management Vitamin D replacement (e.g. 1α-hydroxycholecalciferol).

Paget's disease

Increased bone turnover with disorganized new bone formation.

Aetiology Unknown.

Clinical features

Bone pain and deformity may be present.

Often an incidental finding on X-ray.

Common sites Pelvis, long bones, lumbar spine, skull.

Investigation X-ray shows osteolytic and osteosclerotic areas with expansion of bone and coarse trabeculation.

Alkaline phosphatase is increased. Plasma calcium and phosphate are normal.

Management

Analgesia.

Diphosphonates (e.g. disodium etidronate) prevent osteoclastic activity, but should not be given for courses of longer than 3 months.

Calcitonin inhibits bone resorption and turnover.

HAEMATOLOGY

Anaemia (see p. 243)

Leukaemias

Malignant proliferation of blood-forming cells. Broadly classified according to whether lymphocytic or myeloid (marrow-related) cell lines are involved, and whether the disease untreated is likely to follow an acute, rapidly fatal, or more prolonged chronic course.

Clinical features

Acute lymphatic leukaemia Commonest form of childhood leukaemia. Infiltration of bone marrow with lymphoblastic cells causes anaemia, bruising (thrombocytopenia) and infections (neutropenia).

Lymphoblasts are usually present in the peripheral blood and always in the marrow. Lymphadenopathy, splenomegaly and hepatomegaly occur.

Chronic lymphatic leukaemia Occurs in the elderly. Generalized lymphadenopathy. Raised white cell count with lymphocytosis. Usually follows a benign course — treatment only indicated if symptoms develop.

Acute myeloid leukaemia All ages but less common in childhood. Myeloblasts infiltrate the marrow and are found in the blood. Anaemia, bleeding or infections are common. Involvement of other organs is unusual.

Chronic myeloid leukaemia Usually presents in middle age, often insidiously with anaemia, weight loss and fever. White cell count is markedly raised with myeloid precursors in the marrow and peripheral blood. The spleen and, in later stages, the liver are markedly enlarged.

In over 90% of patients leucocytes contain the Philadelphia chromosome, a translocation of the long arm of chromosome 22 to chromosome 9.

Management

Supportive treatment with transfusions and antibiotics.

Cytotoxics (destroy rapidly dividing cells) alone or in combination with radiotherapy.

In some cases induction of remission by intensive chemotherapy is followed by bone marrow transplantation.

Treatment of leukaemia is under continuous review, and many patients are entered into multi-centre trials.

Lymphoma

Solid tumours of the lymphoreticular system. Divided histologically into two main types — Hodgkin's disease, characterized by the presence of multi-nucleated giant cells (Reed–Sternberg cells), and non-Hodgkin's lymphoma.

Symptoms Lethargy, anorexia, weight loss, fever, night sweats, pruritus.

Signs Painless lymphadenopathy. Hepatomegaly and splenomegaly may occur.

Diagnosis Usually made on lymph node biopsy.

Treatment Chemotherapy, radiotherapy or a combination of the two, depending on clinical, radiological and histological staging.

Myeloma

Malignant proliferation of a specific clone of plasma cells, resulting in the production of a monoclonal immunoglobulin known as a paraprotein.

Clinical features

General Malaise, lethargy, weight loss.

Bone destruction From the expanding plasma cell clone causes pain, fractures and hypercalcaemia.

Investigation

Anaemia with raised ESR.

Monoclonal antibody detected as discrete 'M' band on plasma protein electrophoresis.

Free immunoglobulin light chains may be detectable in the urine as Bence-Jones protein (precipitates on heating to 56°C, redissolves on boiling).

Osteolytic lesions on X-ray.

Renal failure may result from paraprotein deposition in the kidneys or hypercalcaemia.

Management Chemotherapy with cytotoxic drugs. Painful bone lesions may respond to radiotherapy.

Coagulation disorders (see p. 250).

INFECTIONS

Influenza

An acute viral infection.

Major features

Acute onset.

Fever and shivers/rigors.

Headache.

Muscle and joint aching.

Cough and sore throat.

Viral types

Type A (Asian flu) — widespread epidemics and pandemics.

Type B — localized outbreaks.

Type C — sporadic cases.

Strains Distinguished by characteristic haemagglutinin and neuraminidase.

Management

Fluids by mouth.

Aspirin or paracetamol to reduce temperature and relieve pain.

Prevention Active immunization for the elderly and those with chronic heart or lung disease, and for medical staff in pandemics.

NB: Major complication: staphylococcal pneumonia during some epidemics.

Mumps

An acute viral (paramyxovirus) infection — spread by droplets of saliva; there is no rash in mumps.

Clinical features

Acute onset of fever.

Painful swelling of parotid and other salivary glands.

Orchitis (15%) and oöphoritis (5%).

Rarely meningitis, deafness, pancreatitis.

Management

Prevent by immunization (mumps, measles, rubella (MMR) vaccine).

Treat by high fluid intake, paracetamol for pain and fever.

Isolation If in hospital for 9 days after onset of salivary gland swelling (roughly until the swelling goes).

Measles

Acute, highly infectious and communicable paramyxovirus infection. Miserable child with runny eyes, runny nose and blotchy rash.

Clinical features

Acute onset.

Fever and misery.

Conjunctivitis, sinusitis and cough.

Rash — red, blotchy facial rash (days 3–4) spreading to cover entire body (days 4–7). Koplik's spots in buccal mucosa, i.e. 'grains of sand inside cheeks', are diagnostic.

Rarely encephalitis.

Management

Prevent by immunization (MMR vaccine).

Treat symptomatically — fluids.

Paracetamol for pain and fever.

Isolation Away from school until 4 days after rash appears.

Chickenpox and zoster

Caused by herpes varicella-zoster virus.

Chickenpox

Clinical features

Acute febrile illness, more severe in adults.

Skin rash — macular (flat) and papular (slightly raised) red lesions becoming, over a few hours, vesicular (blisters), which last 3—4 days. The vesicles may become infected (pustules), and also scab.

The vesicles appear in crops.

Rarely, acute pneumonia and staphylococcal septicaemia.

Communicability

Droplet respiratory spread 2 days before rash.

By direct contact with vesicles until they crust.

Isolation

Away from school until vesicles disappear.

Strict isolation if in hospital as danger of spread to ill and immunosuppressed patients.

Management

Supportive.

Specific immune globulin for neonates of infected mothers, very ill contacts and patients on immunosuppressive agents (steroids, cytotoxics).

Acyclovir intravenously to the immunosuppressed.

Herpes zoster (shingles)

Aetiology Following chickenpox the virus remains dormant in dorsal root ganglia until reactivation occurs. This is not uncommon in otherwise healthy people, but may be due to diminished resistance in immunocompromised or debilitated patients.

Clinical features Pain precedes the lesions, which are localized to a single spinal or cranial sensory ganglion. Vesicles are grouped on an inflamed base along sensory nerve route distribution (zoster = band or girdle). Any nerve may be involved, including the ophthalmic division of the fifth nerve (the eruption involves the cornea). Motor nerve roots may also be affected (in the Ramsay Hunt syndrome the geniculate ganglion of the facial nerve (p. 121) is affected, causing facial palsy with herpetic vesicles in the external auditory meatus).

Isolation Lesions are infectious — patients should be isolated from the non-immune and immunocompromised.

Complications

Secondary bacterial infection.

Corneal scarring if the ophthalmic division of the trigeminal nerve is affected.

Post-herpetic neuralgia — pain at the site of healed lesions, almost universally associated with depression.

Management

Acyclovir (topical or oral) may help if given early, and may reduce the incidence of post-herpetic neuralgia.

Intravenous acyclovir is usually required in the immunocompromised.

If cornea involved, hydrocortisone to prevent corneal scarring and atropine to dilate pupil and prevent fibrosis between iris and lens.

Local anaesthetic or alcohol injections into dorsal root ganglion or peripheral nerve may be required for post-herpetic neuralgia.

Herpes simplex

Aetiology Transmission is from direct contact of infected lesions via skin or mucous membranes.

Clinical features Herpes simplex virus (HSV) type 1 usually causes cold sores, whilst HSV type 2 causes genital herpes. Following primary infection the virus remains latent (most commonly in trigeminal or sacral nerves), and may be reactivated, producing recurrent lesions.

Immunocompromised patients may develop systemic infection involving many organs, including the liver (hepatitis) and brain (encephalitis).

Management

Oral and genital lesions are self-limiting but can cause marked discomfort.

Topical acyclovir reduces the severity and duration of lesions.

Systemic infection should be treated with IV acyclovir.

Hepatitis

Inflammation of the liver, most commonly with acute infectious hepatitis A or B but also with hepatitis C, infectious mononucleosis and associated with septicaemia. Always consider the possibility of drug- (including alcohol) induced hepatitis.

Hepatitis A

Aetiology Enterovirus; faecal−oral transmission. Incubation 2−6 weeks

Symptoms Fever, malaise, anorexia, nausea and vomiting, upper abdominal discomfort.

Signs Tender hepatomegaly, jaundice (urine becomes dark and stools pale as a result of intrahepatic cholestasis); occasionally splenomegaly and lymphadenopathy.

Investigation Liver function shows 'hepatitic picture' (raised bilirubin with marked increase in transaminases and mild−moderate increase in alkaline phosphatase).

Leucopenia with relative lymphocytosis.

Diagnosis Positive IgM hepatitis A antibody confirms the diagnosis.

Management Rest and abstinence from alcohol whilst spontaneous recovery occurs (no carrier state exists and chronic liver disease never develops). Isolate if hospitalized (infectivity lasts 1−2 weeks after appearance of jaundice).

Fulminant hepatic failure is an extremely rare complication − refer to liver centre for support and consideration of hepatic transplantation.

Prevention Immunize travellers with formaldehyde inactivated hepatitis A virus.

Hepatitis B

Aetiology Spread by infected blood (IV drug abusers) or secretions (sexual contact, particularly homosexuals). Incubation 2−6 months.

Clinical features As for hepatitis A. Arthralgia and skin rashes are common.

Investigations Liver function shows hepatitic picture as with hepatitis A.

Diagnosis Hepatitis B virus has three different antigens (molecules which induce production of an antibody): a surface antigen (HepBsAg), a core antigen (HepBcAg) and an internal component (HepBeAg).

HepBsAg appears in the blood about 6 weeks after acute infection and has usually gone by 3 months.

HepBeAg occurs at a similar time and denotes high infectivity.

HepBcAg is usually found only in the liver. The development of antibodies to HepBsAg usually follows acute infection and indicates immunity. In about 5% antibodies do not appear and HepBsAg persists in the blood (carrier state).

Management Isolate if hospitalized. In the majority of cases spontaneous recovery occurs and treatment is supportive, as for hepatitis A.

The carrier state is usually asymptomatic but is associated with chronic hepatitis and hepatocellular carcinoma. Treatment with interferon may reverse HepBsAg carriage.

Prevention Vaccinate high-risk groups with recombinant HepBsAg.

Delta agent The delta agent is a defective ribonucleic acid (RNA) virus which depends on the hepatitis B virus to replicate. It can cause recurrent hepatitis in HepBsAg-positive patients. Chronic infection is usually associated with progressive liver disease.

Hepatitis C

Aetiology Parenterally transmitted (IV drug abusers, contaminated blood products) small RNA virus.

Clinical features Similar to hepatitis B. It is associated with chronic hepatitis.

Tuberculosis

Aetiology

Infection with *Mycobacterium tuberculosis* predominantly affecting:
- lungs;
- lymph nodes and reticuloendothelial system.

Less commonly:
- kidney;
- brain;
- bones;
- pericardium.

Pulmonary

Clinical features

Fever.

Anorexia and weight loss.

Cough.

Sputum with haemoptysis.

Diagnosis

Stain sputum for acid- and alcohol-fast bacilli.

CXR changes of bronchopneumonia — usually upper lobes.

Lymphoreticular

Clinical features

Fever.

Anorexia and weight loss.

Isolated 'cold' node in neck or generalized.

Lymph node enlargement.

Enlargement of liver and spleen.

Diagnosis Histology and culture of lymph node or liver biopsy.

Treatment

Isolate 'open' (sputum-positive) cases for 1–2 weeks after starting antibiotics.

Antibiotic therapy with a combination of three agents (all have side effects) until sensitivity known (culture takes 4–7 weeks).

Usually:

• rifampicin (hepatic enzyme induction, may progress to hepatitis; colours saliva and urine secretions orange);

• isoniazid (peripheral neuritis; hepatitis);

• pyrazinamide (hepatitis) or ethambutol (optic neuritis).

Prevention Vaccinate with Bacillus Calmette-Guérin (BCG) — live attenuated strain of TB.

Acquired immunodeficiency syndrome (AIDS)

Aetiology Infection with human immunodeficiency virus (HIV) by:

• intercourse — anal or vaginal;

• intravenous injection — drug addicts;

• contaminated blood products — haemophiliacs.

Clinical features

Anorexia and weight loss.

Fever.

Generalized lymph node enlargement.

Malignancies, including Kaposi's sarcoma (usually skin).

Opportunistic infections (Table 3.1).

Pulmonary Pneumonia — CMV, pneumocystis and TB.

CNS Meningitis, encephalitis, choroidoretinitis — toxoplasma, cryptococcal, herpes simplex, CMV.

Abdominal Diarrhoea — cryptosporidial.

Other fungal and viral infections Candida, *Aspergillus*, herpes zoster.

Communicable Diseases Centre (CDC) classification

Group I   Acute seroconversion (may be febrile illness).

Group II   Asymptomatic infection.

Group III Persistent generalized lymphadenopathy.

Group IV   AIDS and AIDS-related complex (ARC) grouped according to: (i) constitutional disease (ARC) (e.g. fever, weight loss, diarrhoea); (ii) neurological disease; (iii) secondary infection; (iv) secondary malignancy; (v) other conditions.

Investigations

Reduced cluster of differentiation 4 (CD4) lymphocyte count.

HIV antibodies.

Management

Counselling — before and after diagnosis.

Azidothymidine (AZT) to inhibit viral reverse transcriptase.

Treatment of opportunistic infections.

Table 3.1 Common opportunistic infection of AIDS and the therapy of choice

Common treatable opportunistic infections	Therapy of choice	Prophylaxis
Pneumocystis carinii pneumonia	Pentamidine by inhalation or Septrin	Pentamidine or Septrin
Toxoplasmic encephalitis	Pyrimethamine + sulphadiazine	Nil
Cryptococcal meningitis	Amphotericin B + 5-flucytosine or fluconazole	Fluconazole
Cytomegalovirus	Ganciclovir or foscarnet	Ganciclovir or foscarnet
Herpes simplex and zoster	Acylovir	
Mycobacterial TB	Standard TB therapy	

Infections of travellers

Acute infections of travellers returning especially from the tropics include:

- malaria;
- typhoid;
- *Salmonella*, amoebic and *Giardia* dysentery.

TB and venereal diseases occur worldwide.

Malaria

An acute parasitic (*Plasmodium falciparum*, *P. malariae*, *P. ovale* and *P. vivax*) infection transmitted in blood by the bite of the female anopheline mosquito.

Clinical features

Acute onset.

Swinging fever with hot and cold chills and rigors.

Splenomegaly.

Cerebral and renal complications in malignant tertian malaria (*P. falciparum*).

Diagnosis
Parasites seen in red blood cells (RBCs) on examination of blood films.

NB: If the parasitaemia is very low they may be easily missed — this does not exclude the diagnosis.

Management

Prevention — mosquito netting to houses and for sleep.

Cover ankles and wrists at sunset.

Proguanil and chloroquine (and Maloprim for Southeast Asia).

Treatment
Quinine by mouth or intravenously if very ill or nauseated.

Primaquine to eradicate liver phase if *P. ovale* or *P. vivax*.

Typhoid

A bacterial infection from *Salmonella typhi*, usually confined to the gut, but may spread to the blood to cause bacteraemia.

Clinical features
Gradual onset within 21 days of return and with:

- headache and malaise;
- vague abdominal pain;
- cough and constipation.

Later features (second week) include persistent fever, abdominal distension, diarrhoea, rose spots on upper abdomen.

Later still (third week): delirium, coma and death.

Investigations

Stool for culture.

Blood for culture on suspicion of typhoid.

The WBC is typically normal or low.

Management

Isolation to prevent spread.

Rehydration to maintain fluid balance and renal function.

Antibiotics (ciprofloxacin or cefotaxime).

Gastroenteritis

Usually diarrhoea.

Aetiology

Often cause never found (presumed viral or *Escherichia coli*).

Salmonella (bacillary) dysentery.

Amoebic dysentery.

Giardia lamblia.

Home-grown dysentery:

- viral;
- *E. coli*;
- *Salmonella*;
- *Campylobacter*.

Investigations

Stools for organisms — microscopy and culture.

Blood cultures if patient systemically unwell.

Management

Isolate in hospital until organism known.

Rehydration — oral or intravenous.

Specific antimicrobial therapy when organism identified:

- *Salmonella* — trimethoprim/ampicillin;
- *Amoeba* — metronidazole;
- *Giardia* — metronidazole.

4 Emergencies

4

LIFE-THREATENING CONDITIONS

This chapter deals with the major clinical features and key therapeutic action of life-threatening conditions.

Acute laryngeal obstruction

Clinical features

Acute breathlessness.

Inspiratory croak (stridor).

Indrawing of intercostal muscles on inspiration.

Aetiology

Inhalation of foreign body — peanut, lump of meat.

Acute epiglottitis in infants (infection with *Haemophilus influenzae*).

Angio-oedema — oedematous swelling of the eyes, mouth, respiratory tract as part of an allergic response (or more rarely a familial condition).

Management
Inhaled body: removal

- Open mouth;
- Heimlich manoeuvre — grasp the patient from behind and exert sudden pressure in the epigastrium directed upward through the diaphragm (a modified bear hug).

Acute epiglottitis

- Do not attempt to look at epiglottis — may precipitate complete obstruction;
- tracheal intubation by anaesthetist or ear, nose and throat (ENT) surgeon if almost complete;
- antibiotics (e.g. cefotaxime intravenously (IV)).

Angio-oedema

- Adrenaline 1 ml 1 : 1000 intramuscularly (IM) or subcutaneously.

NB: Emergency tracheostomy in expert hands.

Tension pneumothorax

Clinical features
Progressive dyspnoea.

Cyanosis.

Unilateral chest signs — tracheal shift away, reduced movement, hyperresonance on percussion, reduced breath sounds.

Management
- Insert intercostal drain (insert large IV cannula if desperate).

Severe asthma

Clinical features
Persistent severe dyspnoea — may be too breathless to speak and wheeze may be absent if very little air is moving in airways.

Exhaustion.

Cyanosis.

Tachycardia and pulsus paradoxus.

Unable to use peak flow meter or peak flow markedly reduced (less than 100 litres/minute).

Arterial gases — reduced partial pressure of arterial oxygen (Pa_{O_2}), increased partial pressure of arterial carbon dioxide (Pa_{CO_2}) and decreased pH.

Management
- Continuous oxygen at high concentration (use nasal cannulae to deliver up to 100%);
- β_2 agonists by nebulizer or intravenously;
- IV steroids;
- IV fluids.

Consider artificial ventilation for progressive respiratory failure.

Severe asthma may develop suddenly and cause respiratory arrest (see cardiorespiratory arrest, p. 231) — never delay treatment whilst awaiting results of investigations; never give sedatives, and always consider the possibility of a pneumothorax.

Pulmonary embolism (massive)

Clinical features A large embolus may lodge in and obstruct the right or left pulmonary artery or the main pulmonary trunk, causing cardiorespiratory arrest.

Management

See cardiorespiratory arrest, p. 231. If resuscitation is successful and the diagnosis suspected on clinical grounds (pp. 174–5), proceed to pulmonary angiography followed by thrombolysis or surgical removal of embolus. There may be time to set up cardiopulmonary bypass.

Acute left ventricular failure (pulmonary oedema)

Clinical features

Severe dyspnoea.
Cyanosis, sweating, cold peripheries.
Copious frothy, blood-stained sputum.
Jugular venous pulse (JVP) raised.
Tachycardia, gallop rhythm.
Crackles at lung bases, wheeze throughout chest.

Management

- Sit patient upright;
- oxygen (100% if no features of chronic lung disease);
- IV frusemide (40–80 mg);
- IV diamorphine (2.5–5 mg).

Hypertensive encephalopathy

Clinical features

Hypertension — usually, but not always, severe (i.e. diastolic blood pressure (BP) over 140 mmHg).
Papilloedema.
Confusion progressing to coma.
Sometimes hemiparesis — often reversible.

Management
- Rarely necessary to reverse BP quickly;
- nifedipine capsule 20 mg chewed.

If no effect:
- hydralazine 10–20 mg IM or slowly IV;
- sodium nitroprusside 0.5–0.8 mg/kg/minute by infusion (adjust as BP returns to normal);
- avoid beta-blockers in case cause is phaeochromocytoma — danger of unopposed alpha-adrenergic effects.

Cardiorespiratory arrest

Clinical features
Sudden loss of consciousness.
Absent carotid and femoral pulses.
Respiratory arrest follows shortly after.

Aetiology
Almost invariably cardiac arrhythmia (ventricular fibrillation (VF), ventricular tachycardia (VT) or asystole).
Rarely primary event is respiratory arrest (e.g. severe asthmatic attack).

Management
- Watch patient for 1–2 seconds to ensure correct diagnosis (observe for fluttering and opening of eyelids or return of consciousness);
- recheck carotid pulse;
- if absent, call cardiac arrest team and strike sternum hard;
- external cardiac massage and ventilation through Brooke's airway (give one respiration after every five compressions);
- establish intravenous line;
- defibrillate as soon as machine arrives, with 200 J (ensure everyone is away from the bed or trolley).

Continue until the cardiac arrest team arrives, then:
- intubate and ventilate;
- check rhythm on electrocardiogram (ECG) monitor;
- treat according to following chart (box 4.1, pp. 232–3).

Box 4.1

Cardiopulmonary resuscitation (CPR)

Unresponsive

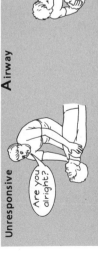

Are you alright?

No breathing

No pulse

Airway

Open airway

Breathing

Rescue breathing

Circulation

2:15

CPR

☎ **Call for help**

Including:
- defibrillator
- airway adjuncts
- oxygen
- emergency kit

Consider
- precordial thump *in witnessed or monitored arrest*

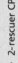

- 2-rescuer CPR

1:5

- mouth-to-mask ventilation

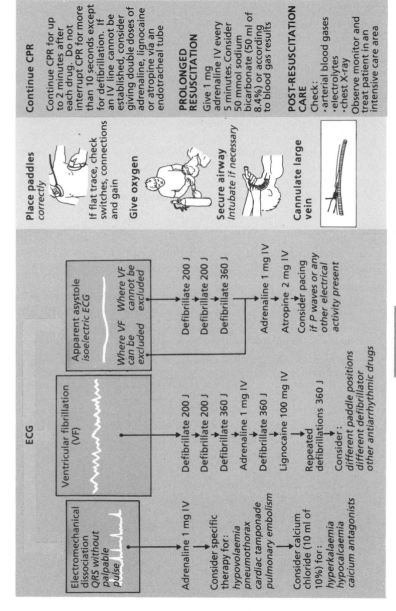

ECG

Electromechanical dissociation	Ventricular fibrillation (VF)	Apparent asystole isoelectric ECG

Electromechanical dissociation QRS without palpable pulse

Adrenaline 1 mg IV

Consider specific therapy for:
hypovolaemia
pneumothorax
cardiac tamponade
pulmonary embolism

Consider calcium chloride (10 ml of 10%) for:
hyperkalaemia
hypocalcaemia
calcium antagonists

Ventricular fibrillation (VF)

Defibrillate 200 J
Defibrillate 200 J
Defibrillate 360 J
Adrenaline 1 mg IV
Defibrillate 360 J
Lignocaine 100 mg IV
Repeated defibrillations 360 J

Consider:
different paddle positions
different defibrillator
other antiarrhythmic drugs

Apparent asystole isoelectric ECG

Where VF can be excluded — *Where VF cannot be excluded*

Defibrillate 200 J
Defibrillate 200 J
Defibrillate 360 J

Adrenaline 1 mg IV
Atropine 2 mg IV

Consider pacing *if P waves or any other electrical activity present*

Place paddles *correctly*

If flat trace, check switches, connections and gain

Give oxygen

Secure airway *Intubate if necessary*

Cannulate large vein

Continue CPR

Continue CPR for up to 2 minutes after each drug. Do not interrupt CPR for more than 10 seconds except for defibrillation. If an IV line cannot be established, consider giving double doses of adrenaline, lignocaine or atropine via an endotracheal tube

PROLONGED RESUSCITATION

Give 1 mg adrenaline IV every 5 minutes. Consider 50 mmol sodium bicarbonate (50 ml of 8.4%) or according to blood gas results

POST-RESUSCITATION CARE

Check:
• arterial blood gases
• electrolytes
• chest X-ray

Observe monitor and treat patient in an intensive care area

4

Coma

Causes
Cardiovascular
  Syncope.
  Cardiac arrest.
Cerebral
  Head injury.
  Stroke.
  Infection (meningitis, encephalitis).
  Epilepsy.
Metabolic
  Diabetes (hypoglycaemia; ketoacidosis; hyperosmolar).
  Drugs.

Management
• Treat urgently for cardiac arrest or suspected hypoglycaemia. Otherwise there is usually time to consider and confirm the diagnosis.
• Roll into the lateral coma position to prevent tongue obstructing the pharynx and to reduce the risk of aspiration pneumonia. *NB*: In self-induced drug overdose and diabetic ketoacidosis aspirate stomach after insertion of cuffed endotracheal tube.

Drug overdose

Management
• Maintain airway and ventilate if necessary (when the patient is severely hypoventilating as assessed by blood gases or, rarely, has stopped breathing);
• remove drug from:
stomach with emetics or gastric lavage (cuffed endotracheal tube if comatose — seek anaesthetic help);
blood by diuretics with urine alkalinization for aspirin, or by dialysis for lithium;
• reduce absorption of drug: e.g. Fuller's earth for paraquat, desferrioxamine for iron, activated charcoal for most other poisons.
Care of comatose patient
Lateral position nursing.

Physiotherapy.

Fluid and electrolyte balance.

Treatment of system failures: cardiovascular, respiratory, renal, liver.

Specific antidotes

Naloxone for opiates.

N-acetyl cysteine for paracetamol.

Desferrioxamine for iron.

Flumazenil for benzodiazepines.

Hypoglycaemia

Clinical features

Usually a known diabetic (look for card in wallet or pocket or Medic-Alert bracelet).

Aggressive confusion progressing to coma.

Sweating.

Management

- URGENT — sugared drink if conscious;
- IV glucose 20—40 ml 50% or IM glucagon 1 mg.

Diabetic ketoacidosis

Clinical features

Usually a known diabetic.

Mild — confusion and irritability.

Severe — coma.

Hyperventilation due to acidosis.

Dehydration due to osmotic diuresis.

Management

- Rehydrate (1 litre of IV saline in half an hour initially);
- insulin (4—8 units IV hourly by infusion);
- empty stomach to prevent aspiration pneumonia;
- replace potassium (whole body potassium usually reduced by 10—25%);
- treat infection if present (often urinary or chest);
- why did it happen?

Toxic hypercalcaemia

Aetiology

Malignant secondary deposits in bone is the most common — carcinoma, myeloma.

Parathyroid hormone (PTH) excess — hyperparathyroidism ectopic PTH secretion (usually carcinoma of bronchus).

Excess vitamin D — self-administered.

Vitamin D sensitivity — sarcoid and other granulomas.

Management

- Rehydrate with IV saline;
- frusemide 40–80 mg IV;
- Bisphosphonates (e.g. IV disodium etidronate or pamidronate).

Tetany

NB: Tetan*us* is an infectious disease caused by *Clostridium tetani*, which causes severe painful muscle spasm. Tetany is muscle spasm due to hypocalcaemia.

Aetiology

Hyperventilation syndrome (metabolic alkalosis).

Hypocalcaemia, usually secondary to surgical removal of parathyroid glands during thyroidectomy, or hypoparathyroidism.

Clinical features

Perioral paraesthesia.

Muscle cramps and spasm.

Convulsions.

NB: Positive Chvostek's and Trousseau's signs.

Chvostek's sign The nerves are excitable and tapping the facial (seventh cranial) nerve branches over the parotid gland produces twitching of the corner of the mouth.

Trousseau's sign Blow a BP cuff up on an arm to over systolic pressure. The ischaemia causes the excitable neuromuscular system of the arm to contract with flexion at the wrist and the metacarpophalangeal (MCP) joints and extension at the proximal interphalangeal (PIP) joints (*main d'accoucheur*).

Management
- Hyperventilation — rebreathe into a paper bag;
- true hypocalcaemia — 10 ml of 10% calcium gluconate IV followed by infusion of 10 ml over 6 hours.

Addisonian (hypoadrenal) crisis

Aetiology
Withdrawal of long-term steroid therapy.
Post-surgical removal of adrenal glands for Cushing's syndrome.
Septic shock (usually patients in intensive therapy unit (ITU)).
Rarely primary adrenal or pituitary failure.

Clinical features
Apathy.
Epigastric pain, vomiting, weight loss.
Hypotension.
Confusion.
Hypoglycaemia, hyponatraemia.

Management
- IV hydrocortisone 100 mg 6-hourly;
- IV saline and glucose.

Thyrotoxic crisis (very rare)

Clinical features Exaggerated thyrotoxic adrenergic features (p. 206) with fever, marked anxiety and sweating, and tachycardia and arrhythmias (atrial fibrillation (AF), VT, cardiac arrest).

Management
- Oxygen;
- beta-blockade;
- dexamethasone to inhibit conversion of T4 to T3 in tissues;
- carbimazole (60–100 mg) followed by;
- potassium iodide (20 mg three times a day (t.d.s.));
(all orally unless hypotensive or shocked).

Sweating is profuse, therefore carefully monitor fluid and electrolyte status.

Epilepsy

Clinical features Persistent grand mal convulsions (p. 194).

Management
- Diazepam (5 mg/minute over 2—4 minutes IV or 5—10 mg rectally) — will control fits in most patients;
- if fits continue, continuous infusion with diazepam or chlormethiazole;
- anaesthetic help should be at hand if continuous heavy sedation is required to control fits.

Haemorrhage

Venous

Bleeding from cuts and abrasions is invariably venous and stopped with light pressure from a clean and preferably sterile dressing. If superficial veins are severed it is sensible to elevate the affected limb to reduce venous pressure, and this is often sufficient to stop bleeding. Nose bleeds will usually stop with steady pressure across the bridge of the nose with the patient leaning forward breathing gently through the mouth.

Arterial

Bleeding from arteries, usually associated with major trauma, is dramatic and treatment urgent. Considerable pressure over the bleeding vessel is required to occlude it proximal to the bleeding site. This is very tiring and it is wise to hand over in turn until surgical help arrives.

Gastrointestinal haemorrhage

Aetiology
Upper gut (all may be dramatic)
  Duodenal ulcer (DU) — 35%.
  Gastric ulcer (GU) — 20%.
  Gastric erosions (stress or non-steroidal anti-inflammatory drugs (NSAIDs)) — 20%.
  Mallory—Weiss oesophageal tears — 10%.
  Oesophageal varices — 5%.

Colorectal

Diverticular disease and ischaemic colitis (these may be dramatic).

Haemorrhoids.

Anal fissures, ulcerative colitis, Crohn's disease and colorectal and caecal carcinoma (these are usually slow and chronic, causing an iron-deficiency anaemia).

Management

• Save life if severe bleeding by replacing circulating volume — monitor with central venous pressure (CVP) line (p. 314); aim to keep at 5–10 cm;

• determine site of bleeding by endoscopy;

• if known chronic liver disease, may be DU, GU or oesophageal varices, but consider urgent endoscopy and sclerosis of varices under direct vision.

With severe or recurrent bleeding seek urgent surgical help, especially in the elderly.

Liver failure

The end stage of chronic liver disease, most commonly from alcoholic hepatitis, chronic active hepatitis or primary biliary cirrhosis.

Clinical features

Aggressive confusion, flapping tremor (p. 135).

Coma (hepatic encephalopathy).

Signs of chronic liver disease

Jaundice.

Spider naevi.

Ascites.

Testicular atrophy and gynaecomastia (in men — reduced hepatic oestrogen metabolism).

Precipitating causes

Infection (usually septicaemia with *Escherichia coli* or *Staphylococcus*).

Gastrointestinal bleed from peptic ulcers or varices.

Alcoholic binge.

Opiates.

Diuretic therapy or drainage of ascites (paracentesis).

Management

- Save life by replacing circulating volume if precipitated by bleeding, and sclerose any varices (use 5% dextrose or blood, avoid saline);
- give thiamine (vitamin B_1) to treat psychosis and confusion in alcoholics;
- remove protein (includes blood) from gastrointestinal tract with lactulose and/or magnesium sulphate enemas;
- monitor fluid and electrolyte balance and renal function;
- check for and treat infection (including ascites for peritonitis);
- check for and treat commonly missed causes of death:
  hypoglycaemia;
  bleeding from vitamin K and clotting factor deficiencies;
  raised intracranial pressure.

Renal failure

Aetiology Consider under three headings: pre-renal, post-renal and renal.

Pre-renal Hypotension from any cause (cardiac, circulating volume loss, septic shock). Initially the kidney diverts the reduced blood flow from the renal medulla to the renal cortex, and acute tubular necrosis (ATN) occurs. ATN invariably recovers (takes days to weeks) if the underlying cause is treated and renal replacement provided. Rarely, prolonged and profound renal hypoperfusion causes cortical necrosis, which is irreversible.

Post-renal Obstruction of urinary tract by:
Prostatic hypertrophy.
Carcinoma — urothelial or compression of ureters from retroperitoneal tumour.
Retroperitoneal fibrosis.
Stone.
Blood clot.

Renal Acute glomerulonephritis, malignant hypertension or end stage of chronic renal disease, secondary to the factors below.
Chronic glomerulonephritis.
Hypertension.
Diabetes.

Chronic pyelonephritis.

Adult (autosomal dominant) polycystic kidney disease in which renal tissue is compressed by multiple slowly enlarging cysts.

Analgesic nephropathy.

Management

The urgent problems are:

- assess circulating volume (clinically or measure CVP);
- replace circulatory volume loss and treat any underlying cause;
- check and monitor fluid balance (weigh daily), urine output, and plasma urea, creatinine, electrolyte and acid−base changes.

Of these a rapidly rising potassium (hyperkalaemia) is the most dangerous and will require urgent treatment with:

IV dextrose and insulin (e.g. 100 ml of 50% dextrose with 20 units soluble insulin) − moves potassium into the cells;

oral or rectal ion exchange resins (calcium resonium);

IV calcium gluconate (protects the heart) whilst renal replacement therapy with haemodialysis or peritoneal dialysis is arranged.

5 Investigations

5

HAEMATOLOGY

Anaemia

Reference ranges (normal values vary slightly between reference laboratories)

Haemoglobin (Hb)

Male (M) $12.5-16.5 \times 10^9$/litre.

Female (F) $11.5-15.5 \times 10^9$/litre.

An automated cell counter (e.g. Coulter counter) gives the following readings:

Haematocrit (packed cell volume (PCV) = volume of red cells per volume of blood)

M   0.42−0.53.

F   0.39−0.45.

Red cell count

M $4.5-6.5 \times 10^{12}$/litre.

F $3.9-5.6 \times 10^{12}$/litre.

Mean corpuscular volume (MCV) 80−96 fl. MCV is haematocrit/red cell count.

Red cell distribution width (RDW) 11.1−13.7. This is an automated measure of anisocytosis: the variability of red cell size.

Mean corpuscular haemoglobin (MCH) 27−31 pg. MCH is Hb/red cell count.

Mean corpuscular haemoglobin concentration (MCHC) 32−36 g/dl. MCHC is Hb/haematocrit. MCH and MCHC are of limited use in the differential diagnosis of anaemia.

Transferrin (iron-binding plasma protein) 2−3 g/litre. Raised in iron deficiency (and pregnancy). Reduced in anaemia of chronic disease, acute inflammation and protein loss.

Ferritin Correlates with tissue iron stores (iron is stored in the tissues in two forms, ferritin and haemosiderin). Only low in iron deficiency states.

A significant difference between one Hb reading and the next is 1 g/dl. If you are attempting to analyse anaemia and are looking at a Coulter-style 'full blood count' (FBC), first check the MCV. See if the cells are normal (normocytic), small (microcytic) or large (macrocytic).

5

Normocytic anaemia

MCV in the normal range. Usually anaemia secondary to chronic disease. It is usually insidious, not progressive and fairly mild (>9 g/litre) except in chronic renal failure. It may become slightly hypochromic and/or microcytic. The white cell count and platelets are normal. The serum transferrin is normal or low but, unlike iron deficiency, the serum ferritin is normal or high (with increased iron stores in the bone marrow). A marrow examination may show malignant disease (leukaemia, myeloma, metastasis) or myelofibrosis.

Anaemia of chronic diseases occurs in:
- chronic renal failure — check serum urea, creatinine, creatinine clearance;
- chronic liver failure — check liver function tests (LFTs), gamma-glutamyl transferase (γGT), prothrombin time;
- connective tissue disease (e.g. rheumatoid arthritis, systemic lupus erythematosus (SLE)) — check erythrocyte sedimentation rate (ESR), C-reactive protein (CRP) (p. 265) and autoantibodies: rheumatoid factor, anti-deoxyribonucleic acid (DNA) antibodies (SLE), anti-neutrophil cytoplasm antibodies (ANCA; present in systemic vasculitis);
- chronic infection (abscesses, tuberculosis (TB), bacterial endocarditis);
- malignant neoplasms.

NB: The anaemia of chronic renal failure can be effectively reversed by treatment with recombinant human erythropoietin.

Microcytic anaemia

MCV is low, e.g. <80 fl. The serum iron is either low (iron deficiency or anaemia secondary to chronic disease) or normal (haemoglobinopathies, usually thalassaemia minor (p. 246)). The spread of red cell size (RDW) tends to be increased in most conditions causing microcytic anaemia, but normal when the microcytosis is caused by chronic disease and thalassaemia minor. The MCH is usually low (hypochromic), i.e. less than 25 pg.

Iron deficiency is due to poor intake, poor absorption, poor iron use by the marrow or increased blood loss (menstrually or from the gut). Check with serum iron (very low) and transferrin, which tends to be high. If in doubt check the serum ferritin (low) and demonstrate low iron stores in the marrow.

Macrocytic anaemia

MCV > 96 and often > 100 fl.

NB: Only perform check tests after full clinical review:
- vitamin B_{12} deficiency (usually pernicious anaemia) — check serum B_{12};
- folic acid deficiency — check red cell folate;
- hypothyroidism — check thyroid function tests;
- liver disease (usually excess alcohol) — check liver function, including γGT.

Check the Hb and reticulocyte response to therapy. If in doubt, marrow examination may provide a definitive diagnosis (megaloblastic). If necessary, when pernicious anaemia has already been treated with vitamin B_{12}, it may still be diagnosed with a Schilling test (B_{12} absorption before and after intrinsic factor).

It is always important to discover the underlying cause of anaemia and to treat it where possible. The peripheral blood film may give extra information.

Peripheral blood film

Reticulocytes (active marrow) — haemolysis or chronic blood loss.

Anisocytes (variation in red cell size) or poikilocytes (variation in red cell shape) — iron deficiency.

Target cells ('Mexican hat' cells) — thalassaemia.

Rouleau formation (clumping together of red cells) — raised ESR (check for myeloma).

Burr cells (irregular 'crinkled' red cell membrane) — renal failure, carcinoma.

Hypersegmented polymorphs — B_{12} or folic acid deficiency.

Howell–Jolly bodies (remnants of nuclear material) — splenectomy (or non-functioning spleen).

Blast cells (immature cells) — acute leukaemia.

Eosinophilia — parasitic infection, allergy, occasionally systemic vasculitis or Hodgkin's.

5

Haemolytic anaemia

The normal red cell life span is 120 days. In haemolytic anaemia premature red cell destruction occurs, predominantly in the spleen, as a result of the factors below.

Intrinsic disorders of red cell

Membrane Hereditary spherocytosis, hereditary elliptocytosis.

Haemoglobin Inherited disorders of haemoglobin synthesis such as sickle cell anaemia (abnormal beta chain synthesis), thalassaemia (deficient or absent alpha or beta chain synthesis).

NB: Thalassaemia causes hypochromic microcytic anaemia with normal iron stores.

Metabolism Glucose-6-phosphate dehydrogenase (G6PD) deficiency, pyruvate kinase deficiency.

Extrinsic factors Red cell autoantibodies (autoimmune haemolytic anaemias), drugs (e.g. methyldopa), hypersplenism.

Released haemoglobin binds to plasma haptoglobins. It is carried to reticuloendothelial cells where it is broken down to iron, globin and unconjugated bile pigments, which are conjugated in the liver and excreted in the stool. Excess urobilinogen absorbed from the intestine is excreted in the urine. Haemolysis is therefore characterized by:

- jaundice with raised unconjugated serum bilirubin;
- increased urobilinogen in urine and stools;
- decreased plasma haptoglobins;
- reticulocytosis due to compensatory increased red cell production.

Reticulocytes

Premature red cells in which traces of nucleoprotein remain as fine, reticular strands.

Normal range $10-100 \times 10^9$/litre.

Increased reticulocytes

Reticulocytes are larger than mature red cells, and if increased may cause macrocytosis. They may be increased:

- after loss or destruction of red cells;
- after specific treatment of anaemia (i.e. iron for iron deficiency, or B_{12} or folate for megaloblastic anaemia).

Platelets
Normal range $150-400 \times 10^9$/litre.

Thrombocytosis (increased platelets)
Causes
After haemorrhage, surgery or trauma.
Splenectomy or splenic atrophy.
Inflammation (as part of an inflammatory response).
Malignancy.
Myeloproliferative disorders, e.g. megakaryocytic leukaemia (rare).

Thrombocytopenia (decreased platelets)
Causes
Adverse drug reactions (e.g. non-steroidal anti-inflammatory drugs (NSAIDs), phenothiazines, gold, thiazides).

Autoimmune thrombocytopenic purpura, in which circulating anti-platelet antibodies lead to premature platelet destruction.

Marrow aplasia.

NB: If also anaemic, exclude disseminated intravascular coagulation (DIC) (pp. $251-2$) and prosthetic valve dysfunction.

Polycythaemia (increased haemoglobin)
Polycythaemia may be primary (polycythaemia vera, leucocytes and platelets usually increased as well), or secondary (e.g. due to increased erythropoietin production in hypoxia or renal disease).

Polycythaemia vera
Hb > 18 g/dl.*
Red cell count $7-12 \times 10^{12}$/litre.*
Haematocrit > 0.55.*
Platelets $> 650\,000 \times 10^9$/litre.
White cell count $> 12 \times 10^9$/litre with basophilia.
Arterial oxygen saturation usually normal (92%).
Leucocyte alkaline phosphatase (LAP) score > 100.
Increased serum B_{12}.

* Also present in secondary polycythaemia.

Increased red blood cell (RBC) mass (>36 ml/kg in men; >32 ml/kg in women).

NB: Splenomegaly occurs in 75%.

Erythrocyte sedimentation rate

Measures the rate of sedimentation (in mm/hour) of red cells in a column of anticoagulated blood. Rapid sedimentation (increased ESR) suggests increased levels of immunoglobulins or acute phase proteins (p. 265) which cause the red cells to stick together. A raised ESR is therefore a non-specific indicator of inflammation or infection. It is usually very high in myeloma.

White cells

Normal white cell count: $4-10 \times 10^9$/litre.

Neutrophils

Normal range: $2.0-7.5 \times 10^9$/litre (40-75% of total white cells).

Neutrophilia (raised neutrophil count)

Causes

Acute bacterial infections.

Inflammation, e.g. arteritis.

Acute tissue necrosis, e.g. myocardial infarction, large pressure sores, burns.

Acute haemorrhage.

Leukaemias.

Neutropenia (low neutrophil count)

Causes

Viral infections, e.g. glandular fever, measles, acquired immunodeficiency syndrome (AIDS).

Drug reactions, e.g. carbimazole, chemotherapy.

Blood diseases, e.g. leukaemias, pernicious anaemia, aplastic anaemia.

Lymphocytes

Normal range (adults): $1.5-4.0 \times 10^9$/litre (20-45% of total).

There are two main sub-populations of T lymphocytes which bear different surface markers or cluster of differentiation (CD) antigens. CD8 cells are 'cytotoxic' — their main function is to recognize and kill cells expressing foreign (usually viral) proteins. CD4 cells are 'helper' cells — they help B lymphocytes to differentiate into plasma cells and produce antibodies. The normal ratio of CD4 : CD8 cells is 2 : 1.

Lymphocytosis (raised lymphocyte count)
Causes
> Acute viral infections, e.g. glandular fever, chickenpox, rubella, mumps.
>
> Lymphatic leukaemia.
>
> Vasculitis and drug hypersensitivity.

Lymphopenia (low lymphocyte count)
Causes
> AIDS — a severely depressed CD4 count predicts the onset of opportunistic infections (pp. 223–4).
>
> Ionizing radiation (treatment for malignancy or accidental).
>
> Chemotherapy for malignancy.
>
> Steroid therapy or Cushing's syndrome.

Eosinophils
> Normal range: $40–400 \times 10^6$/litre.

Eosinophilia (raised eosinophil count)
Causes
> Allergies, e.g. bronchial asthma, urticaria, hay fever, adverse drug reactions.
>
> Parasitic infestation of gut or other tissues (muscles, subcutaneous tissues, liver, urinary tract).
>
> Connective tissue diseases, especially systemic vasculitis.

Pancytopenia
> A combination of anaemia, leucopenia and thrombocytopenia is rare. It is due to either reduced production of cells, caused by:
> - bone marrow infiltration: leukaemia, myeloma, carcinoma, myelofibrosis;
> - bone marrow aplasia: idiopathic or drug-induced (e.g. NSAIDs, chloramphenicol, chemotherapy for malignancy);

- severe vitamin B_{12} or folate deficiency;

or increased destruction of cells, caused by:

- hypersplenism;
- autoimmune disease (e.g. SLE).

Bone marrow examination is the most important investigation in distinguishing these causes.

Coagulation

Cessation of bleeding from damaged blood vessels results from:

- constriction of the affected vessel, followed by;
- formation of a platelet plug, followed by;
- activation of the coagulation cascade (Fig. 5.1);
— leading to formation of a stable fibrin clot.

The commonest cause of *abnormal* bleeding is deficiency of platelets (p. 247), which usually causes superficial bleeding into the skin (purpura).

Clotting factor defects

Clotting factor defects may be hereditary or acquired.

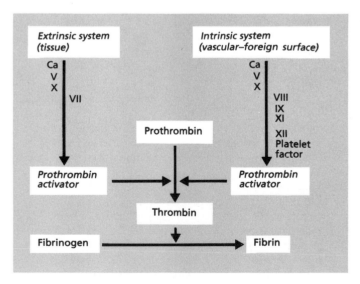

Fig. 5.1 Coagulation mechanism.

Hereditary clotting factor defects Haemophilia A (factor VIII deficiency) and haemophilia B (Christmas disease, factor IX deficiency) are sex-linked recessive disorders of men, carried by women. In von Willebrand's disease (autosomal dominant) factor VIII clotting activity and platelet adhesiveness are both abnormal. Other hereditary defects are extremely rare.

Acquired clotting factor defects Synthesis of factors II, VII, IX and X occurs in the liver and requires the fat-soluble vitamin K as a cofactor. Deficiency may result from liver disease or malabsorption of vitamin K. Oral anticoagulants such as warfarin act as vitamin K antagonists.

Clotting factor defects are investigated by coagulation tests. These are normal in thrombocytopenia.

Prothrombin time (PT) measures the extrinsic system. It is the time taken for the patient's citrated (prevents clotting by binding calcium) plasma to clot when a tissue factor (thromboplastin) and calcium are added (normal 12–15 seconds). It measures deficiencies of fibrinogen, prothrombin and factors V, VII and X. It is prolonged in liver disease and vitamin K deficiency, but is normal in the haemophilias. It is used to monitor oral anticoagulant therapy, when results are often expressed as the INR (international normalized ratio of the patient's plasma compared with an international reference standard; normal is therefore 1.0).

Activated (kaolin) partial thromboplastin time (APTT or KPTT) measures the intrinsic system. It is the time taken for the patient's citrated plasma to clot when phospholipid (a platelet substitute), kaolin (activates factor XII) and calcium are added. It measures deficiencies of factors V, VIII to XII and fibrinogen. It is prolonged in the haemophilias. It is used to monitor therapy with heparin, which inactivates factors VII, IX to XII and thrombin.

Disseminated intravascular coagulation

In severe illness (e.g. septic shock, advanced malignancy, obstetric emergencies), abnormal activation of the clotting system leads to the combination of widespread intravascular coagulation and bleeding due to excessive consumption of platelets and coagulation factors. The platelet count and serum fibrinogen are low and coagulation tests are increased. Fibrin degradation products (FDP) are increased in serum and urine.

Blood grouping and transfusion

Over 400 antigens have been identified on the surface of red cells which together determine a person's blood group. The most important (in terms of their potential for inducing an immune response) are the ABO and rhesus groups.

Naturally occurring antibodies against A or B antigen develop in subjects who lack the respective antigen. Transfusion of incompatible blood into such recipients (e.g. transfusion of group A blood into a group B recipient) leads to lysis of the transfused red cells.

Rhesus-positive patients have antibodies which react with red cells of the rhesus monkey. The strongest rhesus antigen is the D antigen. Patients who lack the D antigen do not develop naturally occurring anti-D antibodies but develop such antibodies if exposed to D-positive blood by transfusion or leakage of D-positive foetal red cells into the circulation during pregnancy. Such antibodies cause haemolysis of D-positive foetal red cells in subsequent pregnancies (haemolytic disease of the newborn).

Hazards of blood transfusion

Transfusion reaction (minimize risk by cross-matching patient's serum with donor blood).

   If clinical manifestations of a transfusion reaction occur (fever, backache, hypotension and haemoglobinuria), stop the transfusion immediately and initiate supportive treatment to alleviate shock.

Transmission of infection (blood is screened for hepatitis B and C and human immunodeficiency virus (HIV).

Circulatory overload (give frusemide with transfusion in patients at risk of heart failure).

Coagulation defects and electrolyte abnormalities (particularly hyperkalaemia — red cell breakdown releases potassium) where large volumes are transfused.

BIOCHEMISTRY

Normal serum values

Sodium	135−146 mmol/litre
Potassium	3.5−5.0 mmol/litre
Glucose	4.0−7.0 mmol/litre
Bicarbonate	22−30 mmol/litre
Urea	2.5−6.7 mmol/litre
Creatinine	60−120 μmol/litre
Calcium	2.2−2.6 mmol/litre
Phosphate	0.8−1.4 mmol/litre
Total protein	62−80 g/litre
Albumin	34−48 g/litre
Bilirubin	<17 μmol/litre
Alkaline phosphatase	25−120 U/litre
Aspartate aminotransferase (AST)	10−40 U/litre
Alanine aminotransferase (ALT)	5−30 U/litre
Lactate dehydrogenase (LDH)	40−125 U/litre
Creatine phosphokinase (CPK)	24−195 U/litre
Uric acid	0.18−0.42 mmol/litre
Osmolality	280−296 mosm/litre

Serum sodium

Increased serum sodium

Serum sodium increased (hypernatraemia) − too much sodium or too little water. Look for signs of dehydration (tachycardia, low jugular venous pressure, postural hypotension, reduced skin turgor).

Check urine sodium (normal 10−20 mmol/litre) and whether urine osmolality is low (<300 mmol/litre) or high (>800 mmol/litre).

The commonest cause is water depletion from:

• *extrarenal loss*:

severe sweating (high temperature, tropics), diarrhoea − urine osmolality high and urine sodium low;

• *renal loss*:

osmotic diuretics (e.g. hyperglycaemia, treatment with mannitol − urine osmolality often normal;

diabetes insipidus (p. 205) − urine osmolality low.

Very rarely it reflects increased total body sodium due to:
- endocrine disease — Conn's (pp. 208—9), Cushing's (p. 207);
- iatrogenic (e.g. dialysis against high sodium dialysis fluid).

Decreased serum sodium

Serum sodium decreased (hyponatraemia) — too little sodium or too much water.

Check serum osmolality and urine sodium.

If serum osmolality is decreased and urine sodium is increased:
- excess renal sodium loss (renal failure, Addison's disease; p. 237);
- inappropriate antidiuretic hormone (ADH) secretion (*NB*: some drugs such as chlorpropamide and carbamazepine can have an ADH-like action on the kidney).

If serum osmolality is decreased and urine sodium is decreased:
- extrarenal loss of sodium (e.g. gastrointestinal tract, burns);
- fluid retention associated with cardiac failure, hepatic failure or nephrotic syndrome.

If serum osmolality is normal:
- usually spurious, e.g. in severe hyperlipidaemia when the amount of sodium in the aqueous phase of plasma is normal, but its concentration is expressed in terms of the volume of the aqueous and lipid phase.

Serum potassium
Serum potassium increased (hyperkalaemia)
Potassium retention
- Renal failure (pre-renal, renal, post-renal);
- decreased mineralocorticoids: Addison's disease, spironolactone (aldosterone antagonist), angiotensin-converting enzyme inhibitors (e.g. captopril, enalapril);
- potassium-retaining diuretics (e.g. amiloride).

Increased supply of potassium Potassium is predominantly intracellular, and released following cell destruction (e.g. haemolysis, trauma, cytotoxic therapy).

Serum potassium decreased (hypokalaemia)

Gastrointestinal losses Diarrhoea and/or vomiting (colonic tumours, particularly villous adenomas, may secrete large amounts of potassium), laxative abuse.

Renal loss

- Diuretic therapy (thiazides, loop diuretics);
- mineralocorticoid excess (renin secreted by the juxtaglomerular apparatus in the kidney converts angiotensinogen to angiotensin. Angiotensin stimulates aldosterone secretion from the adrenal cortex, which causes urinary sodium retention and potassium loss). Causes: Conn's, Cushing's, corticosteroid therapy, ectopic adrenocorticotrophic hormone (ACTH) (tumours), Bartter's syndrome (renal potassium loss associated with juxtaglomerular cell hyperplasia and hyper-reninaemia);
- osmotic diuresis (e.g. uncontrolled diabetes);
- renal tubular acidosis (renal tubular defect associated with potassium loss and an inability to acidify urine – causes: hyperchloraemic, hypokalaemic acidosis).

Shift to intracellular compartment (e.g. insulin therapy, familial periodic paralysis).

Poor intake (including eating disorders, which may be associated with laxative or diuretic abuse).

Serum glucose

Serum glucose increased (hyperglycaemia)

Reduced insulin, resistance to insulin, or increased anti-insulin hormones (corticosteroids, growth hormone, catecholamines, glucagon).

Causes

Diabetes mellitus (World Health Organization (WHO) criteria: fasting venous glucose $>8\,mM$ and/or a glucose of $>11\,mM$ 2 hours after 75 g of oral glucose).

Steroids (therapy or Cushing's).

Acromegaly (increased growth hormone).

Phaeochromocytoma (increased catecholamines).

Haemochromatosis (excessive absorption of iron, which is deposited in skin and pancreas (to cause 'bronzed diabetes'), heart (cardiomyopathy), liver (cirrhosis) and joints (arthritis)).

5

Serum glucose decreased (hypoglycaemia)

Causes

Excess insulin — exogenous insulin in diabetes or sulphonylureas such as glibenclamide (increase pancreatic insulin secretion); acute pancreatitis; islet cell tumour.

Corticosteroid deficiency — withdrawal of long-term steroid therapy; Addison's disease; hypopituitarism.

Liver disease — if diffuse and severe.

Malnutrition.

Alcoholism.

Post-gastrectomy.

Serum albumin

Serum albumin decreased (hypoalbuminaemia)

Causes

Inadequate protein intake — dietary deficiency, malabsorption.

Inadequate protein synthesis — liver disease.

Excessive protein loss — nephrotic syndrome, burns, protein-losing enteropathy.

Liver function tests

'Liver function tests' either measure the ability of the liver to perform normal functions (e.g. serum albumin is a measure of protein synthesis, prothrombin time is a measure of the ability to synthesize clotting factors, bilirubin is a measure of bile salt conjugation and excretion), or measure liver enzymes (alkaline phosphatase, transaminases) which are indicators of liver cell damage.

Serum bilirubin

Bilirubin from red cell breakdown is transported to the liver where it is conjugated to glucuronic acid. Conjugated bilirubin is secreted in the bile and degraded in the gut by bacteria to urobilinogen. Urobilinogen is either excreted in the stool or reabsorbed from the gut and excreted by the kidneys.

Jaundice becomes clinically detectable if bilirubin is >35 µmol/litre.

Causes of increased bilirubin

Hepatocellular failure.

Biliary obstruction.

Haemolysis — chiefly unconjugated and hence acholuric (no bile in the urine).

Gilbert's disease (autosomal dominant) — impaired conjugation of bilirubin. Bilirubin increases on fasting. Other liver function tests are normal.

Alkaline phosphatase

Alkaline phosphatase is found in high levels in biliary canaliculi, osteoblasts, intestinal mucosa and placenta.

Causes of increased alkaline phosphatase
Liver cholestasis
Obstructive jaundice (e.g. stone, carcinoma).

Intrahepatic cholestasis (e.g. drugs such as chlorpromazine, cholangitis, primary biliary cirrhosis.

Obstructive phase of hepatitis.
Bone (osteoblastic activity)
Paget's disease.

Bone metastases (markedly raised if prostatic in origin).

Vitamin D deficiency.

Hyperparathyroidism.

Growth in children (particularly puberty).

Bone fractures.

Normal alkaline phosphatase
Alkaline phosphatase is usually normal in:
- alcohol consumption, unless very excessive;
- Gilbert's syndrome;
- myeloma (lesions are destructive without osteoblastic activity).

Serum gamma-glutamyl transferase
Causes of increase
Increased in liver disease but not bone disease (it very seldom arises from an extrahepatic source). Therefore used to check origin of raised alkaline phosphatase. It is:
- induced by drugs, particularly alcohol (even with moderate intake) and phenytoin;
- increased in liver cholestasis.

Serum aspartate aminotransferase
Increased AST

Active liver cell damage, including hepatitis (viral, drug-induced), metastatic infiltration.

Acute myocardial infarction (peaks at 24–48 hours, may fall to normal by 72 hours). The degree of elevation reflects the amount of muscle damage.

Acute pancreatitis.

Haemolysis.

Serum alanine aminotransferase

This usually parallels the AST.

Muscle enzymes: serum creatine phosphokinase and serum aldolase
Increased serum aldolase and CPK

Muscle inflammation or necrosis.

Acute myocardial infarction – increase starts at 3–6 hours, peaks within 24 hours and often returns to normal by 48 hours. A rise after the fifth day implies reinfarction.

Severe myocarditis.

Polymyositis.

Status epilepticus.

Post-operative.

Burns.

Strokes.

Small rises may follow:
- intramuscular (IM) injections;
- prolonged strenuous exercise;
- direct current (DC) cardioversion.

Cardiac enzymes

The commonly used enzymes are listed below.

CPK (see above) Peak within 24 hours. The CK-MB isoenzyme is more specific to myocardial damage but is also elevated in skeletal muscle disease and muscle trauma.

AST and ALT (see above) Peak 24–48 hours.

LDH Peaks at 3–4 days and remains elevated for 10–14 days. Also released from damaged liver, skeletal muscle and red cells (haemolysis).

Serum calcium

The normal range is 2.2–2.6 mM. Calcium is bound to albumin and 'correction' should be performed when albumin levels are abnormal. For every 1 g/litre that the albumin is lower than 40 g/litre, add 0.025 to the serum calcium (or subtract if serum calcium is raised above 40 g/litre).

Serum calcium increased (hypercalcaemia)
Hyperparathyroidism

Primary Parathyroid adenoma or hyperplasia (in *secondary hyperparathyroidism* increased parathyroid hormone secretion occurs in response to hypocalcaemia, e.g. in renal failure, malabsorption — by definition the calcium is normal).

Tertiary hyperparathyroidism If secondary hyperparathyroidism gets 'out of control', an autonomous parathyroid adenoma develops, causing elevation of both parathyroid hormone and serum calcium.

Malignancy

Bone metastases (commonly breast, lung, prostate, kidney, thyroid).

Multiple myeloma, leukaemia, Hodgkin's.

Secretion of a parathyroid hormone-like factor.

Sarcoid Increased sensitivity to vitamin D — hypercalcaemia often precipitated by exposure to sunlight.

Drugs

Excess vitamin D.

Calcium-containing antacids (milk alkali syndrome).

Rarely thiazides.

Endocrine (rare) Thyrotoxicosis, adrenal insufficiency.

Serum calcium decreased (hypocalcaemia)
Hypoparathyroidism

- Idiopathic;
- post-thyroid or parathyroid surgery;
- pseudohypoparathyroidism (reduced sensitivity to parathyroid hormone).

Inadequate dietary intake of vitamin D or calcium (rarely vitamin D resistance).

Malabsorption.

Renal disease.

Acute pancreatitis.

Serum phosphate

Serum phosphate increased (hyperphosphataemia)

Reduced loss

Renal failure.

Hypoparathyroidism.

Increased load

Phosphate enemas or laxatives.

Excessive vitamin D intake.

Serum phosphate decreased (hypophosphataemia)

Increased loss

Diuretic therapy.

Hypoparathyroidism.

Renal tubular defects (e.g. Fanconi's syndrome — glycosuria, amino-aciduria, phosphaturia, renal tubular acidosis).

Decreased absorption

Malabsorption.

Phosphate binding agents (e.g. antacids such as aluminium hydroxide, calcium carbonate).

Vitamin D deficiency or resistance.

Malnutrition.

Intracellular shift

Diabetes mellitus.

'Refeeding syndrome' (after starvation or severe illness).

Uric acid

Levels of uric acid are labile and show day-to-day and seasonal variation in the same person. They are also increased by stress and fasting.

Serum uric acid increased

Causes

Primary gout.

25% of relatives with primary gout.

Diuretics (particularly thiazides).

Small doses of aspirin (up to 2 g/day).

Renal failure (the level does not correlate with the degree of renal failure — serum creatinine should be used for this).

Increased destruction of nucleoproteins, usually in myeloproliferative disorders — particularly at the start of cytotoxic therapy or radiotherapy.

Psoriasis (one-third of patients).

Uric acid production can be inhibited by xanthine oxidase inhibitors (e.g. allopurinol).

Urea and creatinine

Production rate of urea varies, making it a less useful measure of renal function than creatinine, which is produced at a roughly constant rate proportional to skeletal muscle mass.

Serum urea increased

Decreased excretion Renal failure (pre-renal, renal or post-renal; pp. 240–1).

Increased protein catabolism Steroids, surgery, cytotoxic therapy, trauma, infection.

Increased protein intake Dietary, gastrointestinal haemorrhage.

Serum urea decreased

Decreased synthesis

Extensive liver disease.

Low protein intake (malnutrition or malabsorption).

Increased excretion Pregnancy (glomerular filtration rate (GFR) increases).

Dilution

Inappropriate ADH secretion.

Over-enthusiastic intravenous (IV) fluids.

Serum creatinine increased

Impaired kidney function: 50% loss of renal function is needed before the serum creatinine rises above the normal range; it is therefore not a sensitive indicator of mild to moderate renal injury.

Creatinine clearance provides a more accurate assessment (if performed correctly). The patient performs a 24-hour collection of urine (the first urine passed on waking is discarded, and all urine passed, up until and including emptying the bladder the following morning, is collected). A single measurement of plasma creatinine is made during this time. Creatinine clearance is measured as:

(urine creatinine concentration ÷ plasma creatinine) × urine volume per minute.

In addition to being filtered by the glomerulus, small quantities of creatinine are excreted by the tubules. The creatinine clearance therefore slightly overestimates the GFR. Chromium-51 ethylenediamine tetra-acetic acid ([^{51}Cr] EDTA) clearance more accurately reflects the GFR. It is calculated from the rate of disappearance of a bolus injection of [^{51}Cr] EDTA from the blood.

Serum creatinine decreased
Loss of muscle mass, including muscular dystrophies.

IMMUNOLOGY

Autoantibodies
A number of diseases are associated with production of antibodies against the patient's own tissues. These antibodies can be detected in serum by their ability to bind to purified antigen. Common recognized diseases are listed below with their associated autoantigens. They can be divided into organ specific and systemic.

Organ-specific
Hashimoto's thyroiditis — thyroglobulin, thyroid microsomes.

Graves' disease — thyroid-stimulating hormone (TSH) receptors.

Pernicious anaemia — intrinsic factor, parietal cell.

Addison's disease — adrenal cells.

Diabetes — islet cells.

Goodpasture's disease (lung haemorrhage and glomerulonephritis) — lung and glomerular basement membrane.

Autoimmune haemolytic anaemia — red cells.

Immune thrombocytopenic purpura — platelets.

Pemphigus — epidermal desmosomes.

Pemphigoid — epidermal basement membrane.

Primary biliary cirrhosis — mitochondria.

Chronic active hepatitis — smooth muscle.

Systemic

Rheumatoid arthritis — immunoglobulin G (IgG) (rheumatoid factor (p. 200)).

SLE — double-stranded DNA.

Mixed connective tissue disease — extractable nuclear antigens.

Sjögren's (rheumatoid arthritis, with deficient secretion of lacrimal and salivary glands = keratoconjunctivitis sicca) — salivary gland epithelium, IgG.

NB: There is a tendency for more than one autoimmune disorder to occur in the same individual.

Complement and immune complexes

An inflammatory response to an antigen (e.g. bacteria in septicaemia, autoantigen in autoimmunity) frequently leads to the development of immune complexes (antigen–antibody complexes) and activation of the complement system. (Complement is a series of plasma proteins which, if activated, enhance the removal and destruction of foreign antigens.) Immune inflammatory reactions (e.g. SLE, glomerulonephritis) are therefore characterized by the presence of circulating immune complexes.

Serum complement levels tend to increase during inflammation and infection as part of the 'acute phase response' (p. 265), but are low in immune-mediated conditions and in overwhelming infections due to massive consumption.

The overall complement activity of serum can be measured as the volume of serum (as a source of complement) required to produce haemolysis of 50% of a standard quantity of sensitized red cells (CH_{50} assay).

Causes of low complement

Immune inflammation (e.g. SLE, glomerulonephritis).

Septicaemic shock.

Inherited deficiencies.

If the overall complement activity is low the individual components can be measured.

Inherited deficiencies (of individual complement components) are rare and cause specific abnormalities of the immune response (e.g. recurrent meningococcal infection in C6 and C8 deficiency, angioneurotic oedema in C1 esterase deficiency).

Causes of raised complement
Acute and chronic inflammation and infections.

Cryoglobulins
Cryoglobulins are immunoglobulin proteins that precipitate in the cold. They may be idiopathic or associated with connective tissue disease or haematological malignancies. They may occlude small peripheral vessels (causing digital gangrene) in cold weather.

Detection
Samples are collected into pre-warmed (37°C) tubes and transferred to the laboratory at body temperature, where aliquots are incubated at 4°C, 20°C and 37°C and visually inspected after 24, 48 and 72 hours for precipitation in the 4°C or 20°C samples. Any precipitate should redissolve at 37°C.

Plasma protein electrophoresis
Plasma proteins are separated (according to differences in their electrical charge) into six main bands:
- albumin;
- α_1-globulin (mainly α_1-antitrypsin);
- α_2-globulin (mainly α_2-macroglobulin and haptoglobin);
- β-globulin (mainly transferrin, low-density lipoprotein (LDL), C3 component of complement);
- γ-globulin (immunoglobulins);
- fibrinogen.

Abnormalities
Acute phase reaction A number of plasma proteins increase

dramatically in response to infection or tissue injury (e.g. myocardial infarction). These are collectively termed acute phase proteins, and include α_1-antitrypsin, α_2-macroglobulin and haptoglobin, fibrinogen and CRP (a protein that reacts with the 'C' polysaccharide in the pneumococcal cell wall). CRP is useful in diagnosing bacterial infection (increases CRP) in conditions such as leukaemia and SLE (CRP usually normal).

α_1-*Antitrypsin deficiency* Autosomal recessive; associated with emphysema and cirrhosis.

Paraproteinaemia (p. 216) A narrow dense monoclonal immunoglobulin band (M band), usually in the γ region.

MICROBIOLOGY

In a patient with suspected infection always perform cultures before starting antibiotic therapy. Where the source of infection is unclear, culture urine, blood, and sputum if produced, and perform throat and high vaginal swabs if indicated by history or examination. Always discuss special requirements (e.g. the diagnosis of infection in the immunocompromised) with the microbiology department.

Where cultures are negative, a diagnosis of infection may be made by detecting bacterial antigens or monitoring the antibody response (e.g. detection of meningococcal antigen in the cerebrospinal fluid (CSF) of patients with meningitis, or the presence of IgM antibody, or a rising titre of IgG antibody, against a suspected organism).

Urinalysis

Stick testing of a mid-stream urine (MSU) for glucose, blood and protein should be performed on all patients.

If *glycosuria* — check blood glucose (glucose is normally filtered by the glomerulus and reabsorbed in the proximal tubule — in benign familial renal glycosuria, failure of glucose reabsorption in the proximal tubules results in glycosuria despite normal blood glucose).

If *haematuria* — confirm presence of red cells by urine microscopy.

If *proteinuria* — quantify in a 24-hour collection (normal less than 200 mg/24 hours).

Urine microscopy

Urine microscopy should be performed in any patient with suspected renal or urinary tract disease (including hypertension, subacute bacterial endocarditis (SBE), connective tissue disease — the presence of red or inflammatory cells in the urine may be the earliest manifestation of renal involvement).

Always use a fresh sample of urine, and ask for culture if infection is suspected.

Red cells Bleeding from anywhere in the urinary tract.

White cells Infection or inflammation — organisms may be visible.

Casts Hyaline casts are composed of uromucoid (Tamm–Horsfall protein, which is excreted by normal tubular cells). Cellular casts result from adherence of either red cells (implying glomerular bleeding) or white cells (imply tubular inflammation) to the surface of hyaline casts.

Epithelial cells May be found in normal urine due to contamination by cells from the vulva or prepuce.

Cerebrospinal fluid

Collect three samples into sterile containers (labelled in order of collection), and one into a fluoride tube for glucose (fluoride stabilizes glucose by inhibiting glycolysis). Take a blood sample for glucose at the same time.

Normal CSF is clear and colourless with a pressure of 5–15 cm CSF.

Turbidity indicates either infection, or blood due to:
• stroke (heavily bloodstained in subarachnoid haemorrhage);
• trauma during procedure (turbidity clears in sequential samples).

CSF protein (normal 150–400 mg/litre)

Markedly raised in:
• bacterial meningitis;
• subarachnoid haemorrhage;
• Guillain–Barré (acute post-infective polyneuropathy);
• tuberculous meningitis.

Normal or slightly raised in:
- viral meningitis.
- cerebral abscess.

CSF glucose (normal > 50% of blood glucose)
Reduced or absent in bacterial meningitis.
Reduced in tuberculous meningitis.
Normal in viral meningitis, strokes, cerebral abscess.

White cells (normal < 5 mononuclear cells/mm^3, no polymorphs)
Polymorphs indicate
- Bacterial meningitis;
- cerebral abscess;
- early stages of viral or tuberculous meningitis.

Lymphocytes indicate
- Viral meningitis;
- cerebral abscess;
- tuberculous meningitis.

Red cells

If present consider traumatic tap; numbers decrease in sequential samples.
Small numbers in
- Meningitis;
- cerebral haemorrhage.

Large numbers in
- strokes, particularly subarachnoid haemorrhage.

Xanthochromia

Xanthochromia is a yellowness of CSF supernatant, after pelleting any cells by centrifugation, caused by red cell lysis — indicates that blood has been present in CSF for some time rather than as a result of trauma.

Gram-stain for organisms

The common causes of meningitis are as follows.
Under 5: Haemophilus influenzae — Gram-negative bacilli.
Over 5: Neisseria meningitides (Meningococcus) — Gram-negative intracellular diplococci; *Streptococcus pneumoniae (Pneumococcus)* — Gram-positive diplococci.

Usually lumbar puncture is performed to confirm a suspected diagnosis, most commonly:
  • bacterial meningitis — raised protein, polymorphs and red cells, low or absent glucose, organisms on Gram-stain;
  • viral meningitis — raised protein, lymphocytes, glucose normal, no organism on Gram-stain;
  • subarachnoid — blood-stained, xanthochromia (diagnose by computed tomography (CT) scan if focal neurological signs or signs of raised intracranial pressure).

RADIOLOGY

When looking at any X-ray it is best to check technical factors first:
  • identification — name, date of birth, sex;
  • date of X-ray;
  • side marker;
  • penetration — whether the black/white balance is optimum;
  • positioning.

Check for shadows of normal anatomy. Describe any abnormalities anatomically before attempting to give an explanation. Always compare sides where structures should be symmetrical.

General contraindications to X-rays Remember that X-rays are harmful. Only request an X-ray when there is a reasonable chance that it will affect the management of the patient. Avoid X-rays, unless absolutely essential, if there is any possibility of pregnancy.

Chest X-ray

Indications The chest X-ray is the most commonly requested X-ray. It should be performed in all patients with suspected pulmonary or cardiac disease, and patients with any illness of unknown cause.

Contraindications Nil (see general contraindications).

Procedure The standard view is posteroanterior (PA) (X-rays passing posterior to anterior with the patient's chest against the film), in inspiration (Fig. 5.2). The X-rays are diverging from the source and magnify structures furthest from the film (e.g. vertebrae). An anteroposterior (AP) view (taken if the

Table 5.1 Bacterial and viral causes of meningitis

Organism	Special clinical features	CSF	Microbiology	Antibiotic of choice
Common causes				
Meningococcus	Purpuric rash Septicaemic shock	Polymorphs: $0.5-2.0 \times 10^9$/litre Protein: 1–3 g/litre Glucose: very low	Gram-negative intracellular diplococci Positive blood culture Positive CSF immunoelectrophoresis	Penicillin
Pneumococcus	Cranial nerve damage Otitis media Lobar pneumonia High mortality (10–20%)	Polymorphs: $0.5-2.0 \times 10^9$/litre Protein: 1–3 g/litre Glucose: very low	Gram-positive diplococci Positive blood culture Positive CSF immunoelectrophoresis	Penicillin
Haemophilus influenzae	Commonest in children under 5 years	Polymorphs: $0.5-2.0 \times 10^9$/litre Protein: 1–3 g/litre Glucose: very low	Gram-negative bacilli	Cefotaxime
Coxsackie virus and echovirus	Paralysis (very rare)	Lymphocytes: $0.05-0.5 \times 10^9$/litre Protein: 0.5–1 g/litre Glucose: normal	Positive throat swab Positive stool culture Serum antibody: rising titre	None

Continued overleaf

5

Table 5.1 *Contd*

Organism	Special clinical features	CSF	Microbiology	Antibiotic of choice
Mumps virus		Lymphocytes: $0.05–0.5 \times 10^9$/litre Protein: $0.5–1$ g/litre Glucose: normal	Positive throat swab Positive stool culture Serum antibody: rising titre	None
Rare causes				
Mycobacterium tuberculosis	Subacute onset Altered personality Strokes Cranial nerve lesions Fits in children Pyrexia of unknown origin (PUO)	Lymphocytes: $0.1–0.6 \times 10^9$/litre Protein: $1–6$ g/litre Glucose: low, <1.4 mmol/litre	Acid- and alcohol-fast bacilli Ziehl–Nielsen staining and fluorescence microscopy	See p. 223

5

Leptospira ictero-haemorrhagiae (Weil's disease)	Follows exposure to rat urine (sewers) Associated hepatitis and nephritis High peripheral white blood cells (WBC): $10-20 \times 10^9$/litre	Lymphocytes: $0.2-0.3 \times 10^9$/litre Protein: raised by $0.5-1.5$ g/litre Glucose: normal	Serum antibody: rising titre	Penicillin
Lyme disease *Borrelia burgdorferi*	Associated with cranial nerve lesions (unilateral or bilateral seventh nerve) and assymetrical arthralgia and erythema chronicum migrans	Immunofluorescent antibody tested		Penicillin
Poliovirus	Meningitis (common) Asymmetrical paralysis (rare) Polio incidence increasing with decrease in immunization	Lymphocytes: $0.05-0.5 \times 10^9$/litre Protein: $0.5-1$ g/litre Glucose: normal	Positive throat swab Positive stool culture Serum antibody: rising titre	None

NB: Other rare causes: herpes simplex virus; arbovirus; *Staphylococcus*, *Listeria*, *Pseudomonas*, *Cryptococcus* in immunosuppressed; *Escherichia coli*, streptococci and *Listeria* in neonates.

patient is too ill to stand) magnifies the heart. Lateral views (Fig. 5.3) are used largely for localization of lesions visible on the PA film.

Inspection

Check technical factors first:

The film is incomplete if it does not include the whole of both lung fields, including costophrenic angles, the ribs and surrounding tissues.

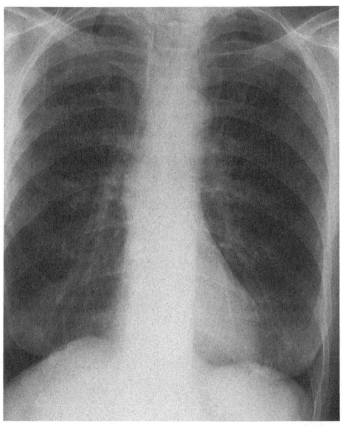

(a)

Check that the film is central. The trachea, suprasternal notch (between the medial heads of the clavicles) and vertebral spines should overlie each other.

Penetration is ideal when you can just see the vertebrae through the cardiac shadow.

Perform a 'free search' for normal structures — bones (ribs, clavicles, vertebrae, scapulae), heart, trachea, bronchi, hila, both breasts, subcutaneous tissue.

Perform a directed search — pulmonary, cardiac, soft tissue.

Directed search
Pulmonary
Lungs Check the density and texture of the lung markings, including the apices (the only markings visible in normal lungs are blood vessels). The costophrenic angles should be sharp. Look for solitary nodules (*carcinoma, metastases, abscesses, granuloma, rheumatoid nodules*), diffuse nodular

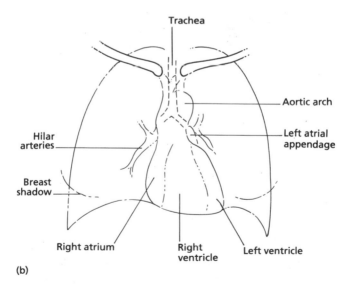

(b)

Fig. 5.2 Normal posteroanterior (PA) chest X-ray. (a) (*opposite*) X-ray; (b) diagrammatic representation.

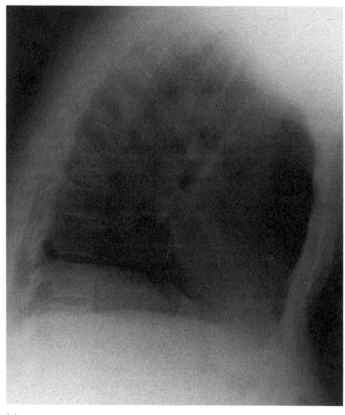

(a)

or reticular shadowing (Table 5.2), or calcification (*TB, chickenpox, histoplasmosis*). Look for areas of consolidation or collapse (Fig. 5.4).

Hila Look for increased hilar shadowing (vascular or enlarged nodes of *sarcoid, TB, lymphoma* or *carcinoma*).

Pleura Examine the pleura for areas of thickening, calcification (*TB, asbestosis, previous haemorrhage*) or effusions (*pulmonary oedema* or *pulmonary inflammation* due to *infection,*

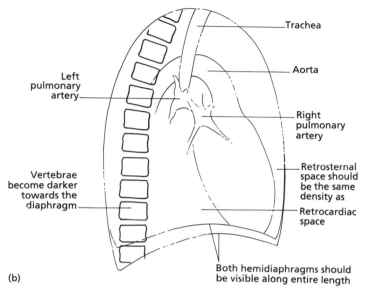

Fig. 5.3 Lateral chest X-ray. (a) (*opposite*) X ray; (b) diagrammatic representation.

infarction, malignancy or *connective tissue disease*). Small effusions cause blunting of the costophrenic angle, larger effusions produce shadowing with a meniscus or curved upper edge. A pneumothorax appears as a fine line, usually parallel to the rib cage, with no markings peripheral to it.

Cardiac

Size The maximum diameter of the heart on a PA film is normally less than half the maximum diameter of the thoracic cage (cardiothoracic ratio less than 0.5). Enlargement of the heart occurs with cardiac dilatation (*heart failure, valvular disease, prolonged hypertension*) or the presence of a peri-cardial effusion.

Left atrial enlargement (due to mitral stenosis) Causes
  • prominence of the left atrial appendage (upper left heart border);

Table 5.2 Common causes of diffuse nodular or reticular shadowing

Cause	Associated radiological features
Pulmonary oedema	Increased heart size, dilatation of upper lobe veins, septal lines
Sarcoidosis	Hilar lymphadenopathy
Miliary TB	Hilar lymphadenopathy, patchy consolidation
Pneumoconiosis	Predominantly upper zones. Opacities of progressive massive fibrosis
Asbestosis	Pleural thickening or calcification
Fibrosing alveolitis	Predominantly lower zones
Lymphangitis carcinomatosis	Septal lines, bronchial wall thickening, hilar nodes

- double contour adjacent to the right heart border;
- elevation of the left main bronchus.

Enlargement of other chambers is difficult to distinguish radiologically.

Main vessels Look for aortic dilatation (*hypertension, aortic valve disease, aneurysm*), which causes a prominent aortic shadow to the right of the mediastinum. Enlargement of the pulmonary artery (*right-to-left shunts, pulmonary hypertension*) produces a prominent bulge on the left border of the mediastinum.

Valves Look for valvular calcification (*rheumatic valve disease*). Pericardial calcification usually indicates old *TB*.

Lung fields Look for evidence of heart failure. Pulmonary venous hypertension causes prominence and dilatation of the upper lobe pulmonary vessels. Pulmonary oedema causes mottling of the lung fields, areas of consolidation and fluid collections, which become visible as pleural effusions or fluid in interlobar fissures or interlobular septa (Kerley B lines).

Bones and soft tissues Look for sclerotic or lytic lesions (p. 294). Examine the diaphragms (right usually 2.5 cm higher than the left), checking for subphrenic air. In women look for both breast shadows. Examine the vertebrae, examining the pedicles, transverse processes and spinous processes (Fig. 5.5).

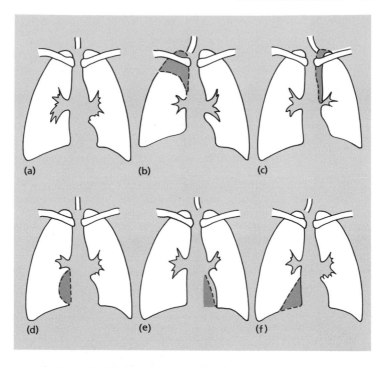

Fig. 5.4 Radiological appearance of lobar collapse. (a) Normal. (b) Right upper lobe: trachea deviated to right; right diaphragm and hilum elevated. (c) Left upper lobe: trachea deviated to left; left hilum and diaphragm elevated. (d) Right middle lobe: right heart border lost. (e) Left lower lobe: trachea may deviate to left; shadow behind heart. (f) Right lower lobe: trachea may deviate to right; outline of right diaphragm lost.

Computed tomography

The presence and extent of mediastinal, pulmonary or pleural masses can be further defined by CT scanning, in which serial axial sections are taken through the thorax (Fig. 5.6).

Isotope lung scan (ventilation perfusion scan)

Indications Suspected pulmonary embolus.

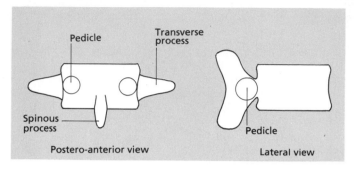

Fig. 5.5 Radiological appearance of vertebrae. *NB*: (i) Destruction of the pedicles usually indicates metastases or myeloma. (ii) Dense vertebrae occur with sclerotic metastases, Paget's disease and malignant lymphoma. (iii) Spondylosis (a result of degeneration of intervertebral discs) causes disc space narrowing and osteophytes.

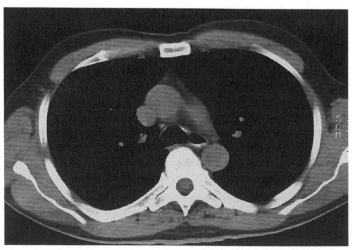

(a)

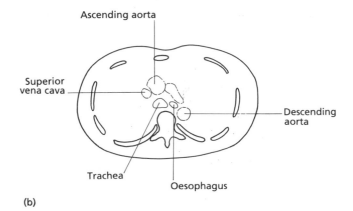

(b)

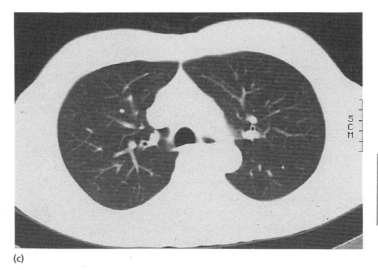

(c)

Fig. 5.6 Computed tomography (CT) of chest. (a) (*opposite*) CT;
(b) diagrammatic representation; (c) the same CT in which a different
window setting has been used to visualize the lung markings (the
window settings determine the range of densities displayed by the
computer).

Contraindications Nil. (See general contraindications.)
Previous abnormal scans should be available for comparison.

Procedure

Perfusion scan Macroaggregates of technetium-99m [^{99m}Tc]-labelled albumin injected intravenously become trapped in pulmonary capillaries, giving a true reflection of blood flow.

Ventilation scan A radioactive gas (e.g. xenon-133) is inhaled.

Inspection Perfusion defects in areas with normal ventilation occur in pulmonary embolism. Matched perfusion and ventilation defects occur in *pneumonia*, *pulmonary oedema*, *airways disease* and *old pulmonary infarcts*.

Plain abdominal X-ray

Indications

Acute abdomen.

Prior to performing intravenous urogram or barium enema.

Contraindications Nil (see general contraindications).

Procedure A supine abdominal film should be combined with an erect chest X-ray when investigating an acute abdomen.

Inspection Look for dilatation of the stomach, small intestine or large bowel. The common causes are: *obstruction, paralytic ileus* or *volvulus* (twisting of the bowel). Dilated small bowel loops are centrally distributed, with valvulae conniventes running across their diameter, which is usually less than 5 cm. In dilated large bowel, haustra do not cross the full diameter, which often exceeds 5 cm. The loops tend to be peripheral and may contain solid faeces.

Look for abdominal calcification (Table 5.3).

Inspect the erect chest X-ray for free gas under the diaphragm (*perforation* or *recent abdominal surgery*).

NB: Soft tissue abnormalities are best defined by ultrasound or CT scan (Fig. 5.7).

Barium examination of the upper gastrointestinal tract

Indications Abdominal pain; dysphagia; vomiting; weight loss; gastrointestinal haemorrhage; upper abdominal mass.

Contraindications Complete bowel obstruction.

NB: Upper gastrointestinal endoscopy allows direct inspection of the oesophagus, stomach and first two parts of the

Table 5.3 Causes of abdominal calcification

Lymph nodes	TB
Vascular	Phleboliths; atherosclerosis, particularly in diabetes or renal failure
Bowel	Faecoliths
Pancreas	Chronic pancreatitis
Gall bladder	Gallstones (20–30% calcified)
Liver	Hepatoma; healed abscess; hydatid cyst
Spleen	Cysts; infarcts; TB
Adrenal	Post-haemorrhage; TB; tumours
Urinary tract	Calculi (90% calcified); TB; carcinoma
Uterus	Fibroids
Ovaries	Cysts (benign or malignant)

duodenum. However, a barium meal should always be performed first if there is a history of dysphagia.

Procedure Prior to performing a barium meal the patient fasts for 6 hours. They then drink barium sulphate whilst radiological examinations of the oesophagus (barium swallow), stomach and duodenum (barium meal) are performed.

The mucosal pattern of the stomach and duodenum is more clearly demonstrated by the use of double contrast (air and barium). In such cases the patient swallows a gas-producing agent (e.g. carbex granules) before drinking barium.

Examination of the small intestine is more difficult, but can be performed by barium follow-through. Delivery of barium to the small intestine can be enhanced by giving metoclopramide (increases gastric emptying) or introducing barium directly into the duodenum through a fine-bore tube.

Inspection

Oesophagus The mucosal surface is normally smooth (Fig. 5.8). Look for defects due to *foreign bodies*, *strictures* or *tumours* (usually irregular).

Oesophageal varices (*cirrhosis of the liver with portal hypertension*) create worm-like impressions. Look for *pharyngeal pouch* (projects backwards and downwards from the pharyngo-oesophageal junction) and *hiatus hernia* (herniation of the stomach through the diaphragm). *Achalasia of the*

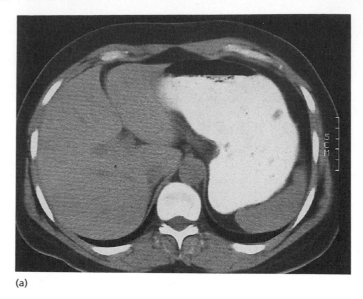

(a)

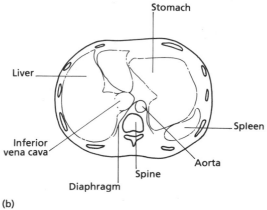

(b)

Fig. 5.7 *(Above and opposite)* CT of upper abdomen. (a) CT;
(b) diagrammatic representation; (c) CT; (d) diagrammatic
representation.

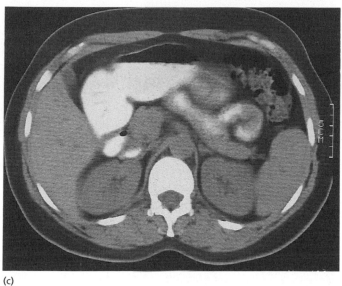

(c)

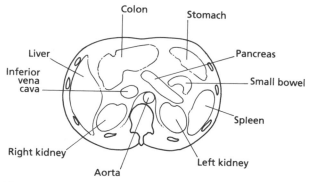

(d)

Fig. 5.7 *(Continued.)*

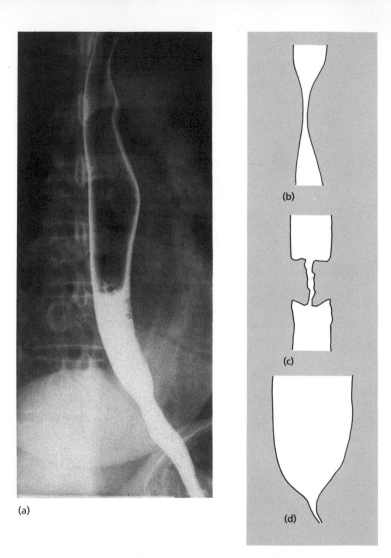

(a)

(b)

(c)

(d)

Fig. 5.8 Barium swallow. (a) Normal barium swallow (X-ray); (b) benign peptic stricture — smooth narrowing, usually at lower end of oesophagus in association with reflux or hiatus hernia; (c) malignant stricture — irregular narrowing with shouldered edges; (d) achalasia — smooth narrowing of the lower end of the oesophagus with dilatation above.

cardia causes a grossly dilated oesophagus, which may contain fluid and food debris.

Stomach and duodenum Ulcers are seen as barium-filled craters. *Benign gastric ulcers* (Fig. 5.9) usually occur on the lesser curve, project beyond the lumen of the stomach and have round regular edges and mucosal folds radiating from the edge of the ulcer crater. *Malignant gastric ulcers* tend to be shallow and irregular, do not protrude into the stomach, are surrounded by irregular mucosal folds and rarely heal in response to treatment.

Malignancy in the duodenum is extremely rare. *Carcinoma of the stomach* may also cause irregular filling defects or infiltrate the gastric wall, causing localized rigidity, progressing in advanced cases to the contracted stomach of *linitis plastica*. Smooth benign tumours (e.g. *leiomyoma*, *fibroma*) also occur.

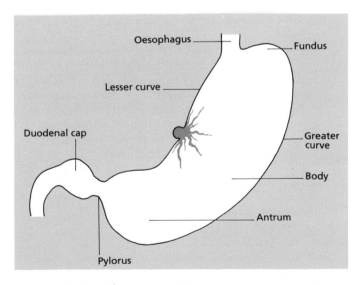

Fig. 5.9 Radiological appearance of benign gastric ulcer. *NB*: Ulcer on lesser curve, projecting beyond the lumen of the stomach, with mucosal folds radiating from the regular edge of the crater.

Small bowel Look for mucosal ulceration or luminal narrowing of *Crohn's disease*, pooling of barium in irregular clumps at the site of an *inflammatory mass* or dilatation in *malabsorption*.

Barium enema

Indications Change in bowel habit; abdominal pain; rectal bleeding; abdominal mass.

Contraindications Toxic megacolon, pseudomembranous colitis and recent rectal biopsy, all of which increase the risk of perforation. Poor preparation of the bowel or the presence of barium from a recent barium meal makes interpretation difficult.

Procedure Adequate clearing of the bowel must be performed, using a low-residue diet, laxatives, enemas, washouts or a combination of these. The patient lies on their side and barium and air (for double contrast) are introduced via a rectal catheter.

Inspection Look for the normal fine mucosal appearance of the colon (Fig. 5.10).

Ulcerative colitis (Fig. 5.11) and Crohn's disease (Fig. 5.12) cause mucosal abnormalities (granular, ulcerated or polypoid appearance) and changes in the configuration of the bowel wall (blunting or loss of haustra, stricture formation).

Look for complications such as fistulae, toxic megacolon (gross dilatation with mucosal islands) and malignancy. Carcinoma may give rise to a localized stricture (apple core appearance) or an irregular filling defect.

Polyps are seen as small round filling defects. Diverticular disease is common in the elderly. The diverticula fill with barium and are seen as outpouchings of bowel. They are commonest in the sigmoid colon.

Intravenous urography (IVU)

Indications Suspected urinary tract pathology. IVU has the advantage of demonstrating the whole urinary tract, but its usefulness has been replaced in many cases by ultrasound, CT scanning and radionuclide scanning. Ultrasound and CT are particularly useful for anatomical studies, and radionuclide

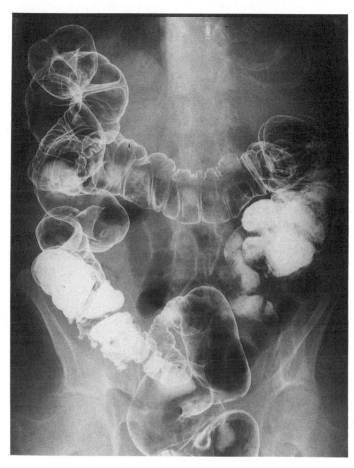

Fig. 5.10 Normal double-contrast barium enema.

scanning for providing functional information.

Contraindications Sensitivity to contrast media. Dehydration prior to the examination should be avoided in renal failure, diabetes or myeloma.

Procedure The patient fasts for 6 hours (unless dehydration is contraindicated). A supine plain abdominal film is taken and

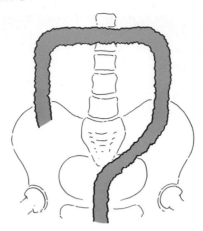

Fig. 5.11 Radiological appearance of long-standing ulcerative colitis. Widespread shallow ulceration leads to shortening and narrowing of the colon.

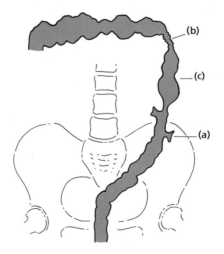

Fig. 5.12 Radiological appearance of Crohn's disease. Patchy involvement of the bowel with: (a) deep ulcers which may lead to abscess or fistula formation; (b) strictures; (c) normal intervening bowel. Areas of disease with normal intervening bowel are known as skip lesions.

inspected to identify the renal areas and look for opacities. Contrast medium is injected as an intravenous bolus and images of the renal areas obtained. A compression band is applied to the lower abdomen to compress the ureters and distend the pelvicalyceal system. The compression is then released and further films taken.

Inspection Timed serial X-rays should be available. First inspect the plain film for renal tract calcification. Contrast is normally visible in the parenchyma as a nephrogram after 1 minute (delayed in renal artery stenosis) and in the pelvicalyceal system by 5 minutes. Measure the size (Table 5.4; normal adult kidneys are 11–15 cm, or three vertebrae in length) and look for the normally smooth outline. An irregular outline due to renal scarring is a feature of *chronic pyelonephritis*, *TB* and *analgesic nephropathy*. The calyces are usually cupped, but become dilated and clubbed (Fig. 5.13) in *urinary tract obstruction* and *papillary necrosis*. Look for filling defects due to *carcinoma*.

After 10–20 minutes the compression bands are removed and contrast should fill the ureters and bladder. Look for

Table 5.4 Causes of small and enlarged kidneys

Causes of small kidneys

Unilateral	Hypoplasia, chronic pyelonephritis, obstructive atrophy, TB, renal artery stenosis
Bilateral	All of above + chronic glomerulonephritis, hypertension, diabetes, analgesic nephropathy

Causes of enlarged kidneys

Unilateral	Compensatory hypertrophy, bifid collecting system, renal mass, hydronephrosis, renal vein thrombosis
Bilateral	Polycystic kidneys, amyloid, acute glomerulonephritis

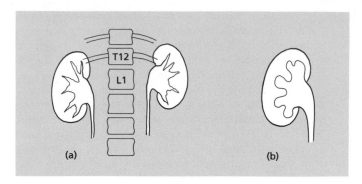

Fig. 5.13 Radiological appearance of intravenous urography (IVU).
(a) Normal IVU; (b) calyceal clubbing.

dilatation due to *obstruction*, or filling defects due to *calculi* or *carcinoma*. Look at the post-micturition film to assess emptying of the bladder and urinary tracts.

Renal ultrasound (Fig. 5.14)

This is useful in determining renal size and contour, in defining the size, location and consistency (solid or cystic) of any renal mass, and in looking for pelvicalyceal dilatation of obstruction.

Isotope scanning

This is most commonly [^{99m}Tc]-diethylenetriamine penta-acetic acid (DTPA) or [^{99m}Tc]-dimercaptosuccinate (DMSA). It can be used to assess renal blood flow, renal function and transit time of filtrate across the parenchyma into the collecting system. It is useful in the diagnosis of renal artery stenosis and urinary tract obstruction. In addition, the renal parenchyma can be visualized for evidence of scarring.

Skull X-ray

Indications Head injury, suspected bony pathology, suspected intracranial pathology.

Contraindications Nil. (See general contraindications.)

Procedure Frontal (20° occipitofrontal and 35° fronto-occipital) views are usually combined with a lateral view.

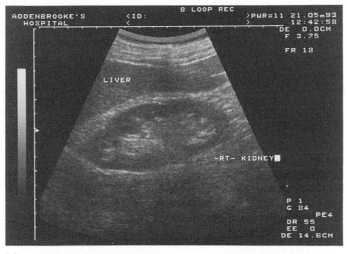

(a)

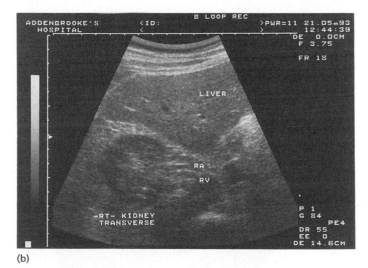

(b)

Fig. 5.14 Ultrasound of the right kidney. (a) Longitudinal scan;
(b) transverse scan.

Inspection Look for intracranial calcification. The pituitary, choroid plexus and intracranial ligaments may calcify normally. Abnormal calcification occurs in tumours, arteriovenous malformations and at sites of previous infection (e.g. abscess, cytomegalovirus (CMV), toxoplasmosis). Examine the pituitary fossa for enlargement due to tumours. Review the bones for fractures and for areas of lysis or sclerosis (p. 294).

Cranial CT (Fig. 5.15)

Indications Suspected intracranial pathology.

Contraindications Nil, although restless, confused or agitated patients may require sedation.

Procedure Serial axial sections of the brain are taken. An intravenous injection of contrast may be given. Increased uptake of contrast (contrast enhancement) occurs at sites of *neoplasm, inflammation* or *ischaemia*.

Inspection Look for enlargement of the ventricles due to *hydrocephalus* or *cerebral atrophy*. Compare the two sides,

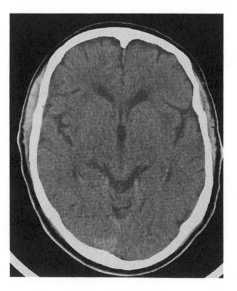

Fig. 5.15 Computed tomography (CT) of head.

looking for areas of abnormal tissue density. High density occurs with *recent haemorrhage, calcification* and *contrast enhancement*. Low density usually indicates *tumours, infarcts* or *oedema*. Look for displacement or compression of structures (mass effect).

Magnetic resonance imaging (MRI) (Fig. 5.16)

MRI is capable of providing high-quality sagittal, as well as axial, sections, and may be extremely helpful in providing further detailed information. It distinguishes white from grey matter, and is particularly useful for identifying lesions in multiple sclerosis. It does not reveal areas of calcification or bone detail.

Skeletal X-rays

Indications Bony injury, suspected bone disease.
Contraindications Nil. (See general contraindications.)
Procedure Views are taken of suspected areas of injury or disease

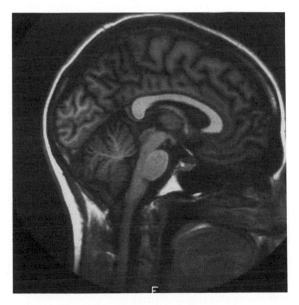

Fig. 5.16 Magnetic resonance imaging (MRI) of head.

(remember that pain may be referred). If generalized bone disease is suspected (e.g. hyperparathyroidism), a limited skeletal survey (hands, skull, chest) may be sufficient.

Inspection Look for areas of increased density due to sclerotic *metastases* or *Paget's disease* (bony sclerosis, cortical thickening, coarse trabeculae and increased bone size). Decreased bone density occurs with *osteoporosis*, *osteolytic metastases* and *osteomalacia* (look for *Looser's zones*, which are linear areas of low density). Examine joints for evidence of *osteoarthritis* (loss of joint space, bony sclerosis, bone cysts, osteophytes) or erosions (*rheumatoid arthritis*, *gout*, *psoriasis*, *ankylosing spondylitis*, *TB*).

Bone scan

Indications Suspected bony metastases or osteomyelitis; to determine whether a lesion is solitary or multiple.

Contraindications Nil.

Procedure [^{99m}Tc]-labelled phosphate complexes are given as an IV injection.

Inspection Look for areas of increased uptake due to tumours, fractures, infection, infarction, Paget's disease.

ELECTROCARDIOGRAMS (ECGs)

Hints and facts (Fig. 5.17)

One little square is 0.04 seconds; one big square is 0.2 seconds. One little square vertically is 1 mV.

Normal PR interval is 0.12 to 0.2 second (three small squares to one big square).

Normal QRS duration is up to 0.12 seconds (three small squares).

The QT interval varies with rate. Upper limits of normal are approximately:

- rate 60/minute: QT 0.43 seconds;
- rate 75/minute: QT 0.39 seconds;
- rate 100/minute: QT 0.34 seconds.

When presented with an ECG, check that it is labelled correctly (patient's name, date, leads for each group of complexes) and then assess the rate and rhythm.

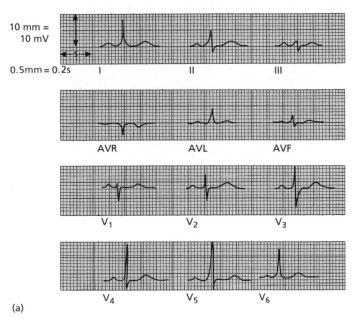

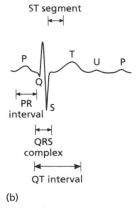

(a)

(b)

Fig. 5.17 (a) Normal 12-lead electrocardiogram (ECG). AVF, augmented voltage F; AVL, augmented voltage L; AVR, augmented voltage R. (b) Waves of the normal ECG.

Rate

Assess the rate by counting the large squares between two QRS complexes and dividing into 300 (i.e. if two squares the rate is 150/minute; three squares 100/minute; four squares 75/minute; five squares 60/minute). If the rate is less than 60/minute the patient has a bradycardia; if greater than 100/minute a tachycardia.

Regularity

Use the edge of a piece of paper to mark off a series of R waves, and then shift the paper along one or more complexes. The marks on the paper will still correspond with the R waves if the rhythm is regular. Total irregularity is almost always due to atrial fibrillation.

Check the mean frontal QRS axis

Use the limb leads, and remember the angles at which these leads 'see' the heart (lead I = 0°; Fig. 5.18). To gain a rough idea of the axis find the lead with the maximum positive deflection (sum of the positive R wave and negative Q and S waves) — the axis lies close to this. Then calculate the total deflection (R wave minus Q and S waves) in leads I and AVF, which are perpendicular to each other (at 0° and 90° respectively). Add these together as vectors (use the squares on the ECG paper) — the net vector is the axis (for examples see Fig. 5.18).

The normal range is 0–90°.

Causes of axis deviation

Left Left ventricular (LV) strain or hypertrophy (e.g. hypertension, aortic stenosis), ostium primum atrial septal defect.

Right Right ventricular (RV) strain or hypertrophy (e.g. pulmonary embolus, chronic lung disease, pulmonary valve stenosis), ostium secundum atrial septal defect (ASD).

Check individual waves in order (i.e. P wave, PR interval, QRS complex, ST segment, QT interval, T wave) for their presence, shape and duration. This always needs to be performed for each lead in turn, although you will come to recognize certain patterns (e.g. bundle branch block, myocardial infarction). It is usually safe to ignore AVR.

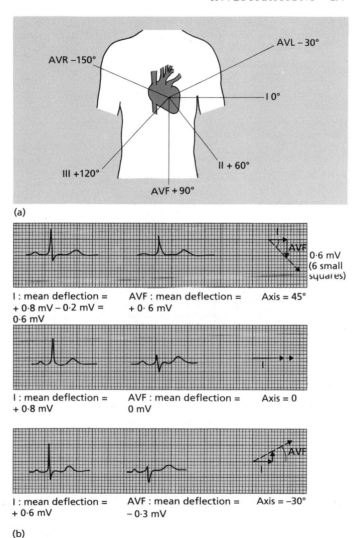

(a)

I : mean deflection = +0·8 mV − 0·2 mV = 0·6 mV

AVF : mean deflection = +0· 6 mV

Axis = 45°

I : mean deflection = + 0·8 mV

AVF : mean deflection = 0 mV

Axis = 0

I : mean deflection = + 0·6 mV

AVF : mean deflection = − 0·3 mV

Axis = −30°

(b)

Fig. 5.18 (a) Position of the limb leads; (b) calculation of the cardiac axis.

P wave (atrial depolarization)

Most easily seen in V_1 and V_2. It is: peaked in right atrial hypertrophy, and bifid in left atrial hypertrophy (left atrial depolarization occurs slightly later than right, giving a second peak); may be 'lost' (in the QRS complex) in nodal rhythm (originates from the atrioventricular (AV) node).

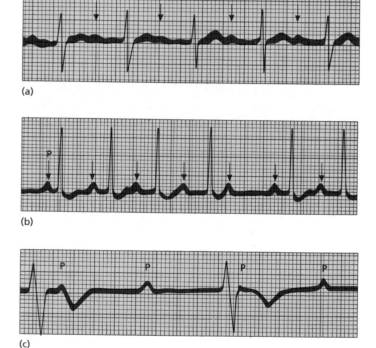

(a)

(b)

(c)

Fig. 5.19 (a) First-degree heart block. PR interval 0.30 seconds. (b) Second-degree heart block (Wenckebach or Möbitz type I). (c) Third-degree heart block (complete). AV dissociation.

PR interval

If the PR interval is longer than 0.2 seconds (one large square), first-degree heart block is present (Fig. 5.19a).

If the normal 1 : 1 ratio of P : QRS complexes is lost but a relationship between P waves and QRS complexes still exists, second-degree heart block is present. The relationship may be either progressive lengthening of the PR interval until one QRS complex is dropped (Möbitz type I or Wenckebach) (Fig. 5.19b) or dropped QRS complexes without a change in the PR interval.

If there is complete dissociation between P waves and QRS complexes, third-degree heart block (Fig. 5.19c) exists. The QRS complex rate (and hence ventricular rate) is usually slow (15–50/minute) and regular. Cardiac pacing is often required.

A short PR interval occurs in the Wolff–Parkinson–White syndrome, in which an abnormal AV conduction pathway (bundle of Kent) predisposes to arrhythmias. The PR interval is short and the QRS complex slurred by a delta wave at the beginning.

QRS complex (ventricular depolarization)

If the QRS complex is longer than 0.12 seconds (three small squares), bundle branch block exists. In left bundle branch block the complex is negative (V- or W-shaped) in V_1 (Fig. 5.20). In right bundle branch block the complex is positive (M-shaped) in V_1 (Fig. 5.21).

Pathological (broad, deep) Q waves are greater than 0.04 seconds (1 small square) wide and greater than 0.2 mV (two small squares deep). They may be normal in AVR or V_1. In the absence of bundle branch block, ventricular rhythms and the Wolff–Parkinson–White syndrome, they indicate myocardial infarction. The site of such pathological Q waves indicates the site of the myocardial infarction – inferior if in AVF, III (the inferior leads – Fig. 5.22), anterior if in the chest leads (Fig. 5.23).

ST segment

The ST segment is depressed in myocardial ischaemia (Fig. 5.24), digoxin therapy and LV hypertrophy.

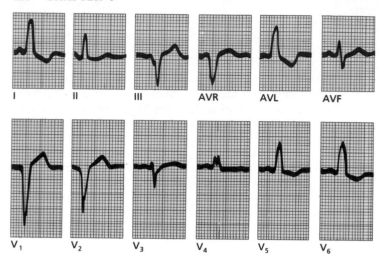

Fig. 5.20 Left bundle branch block. RSR (M-shaped QRS complex)
visible in some of the left ventricular leads, I, AVL and V_{4-6}; and
notched QS complexes in the right ventricular lead, V_{1-2}.

It is raised in myocardial infarction (convex or domed) (Figs
5.22 & 5.23) and pericarditis (concave) (Fig. 5.25).

T wave repolarization

The T wave is peaked in hyperkalaemia (p. 309) and sometimes
acutely in myocardial infarction.

It is inverted in ventricular strain or hypertrophy, myocardial
ischaemia and infarction (as with myocardial infarction, the
leads indicate the site), bundle branch block, digoxin therapy
and cardiomyopathies (abnormalities of cardiac muscle, which
may be ischaemic, drug or alcohol, familial or idiopathic in
origin).

U wave

Follows the T wave and can be present normally. It is increased
in hypokalaemia (see below).

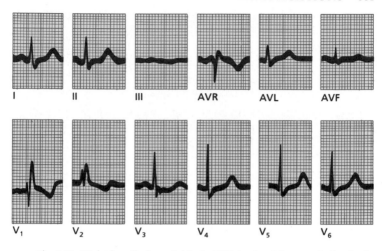

Fig. 5.21 Right bundle branch block. RSR in the right ventricular leads V_{1-2} and slurred S waves in the left ventricular leads I, AVL and V_{4-6}.

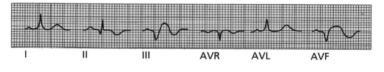

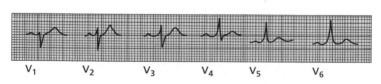

Fig. 5.22 Inferior myocardial infarction.

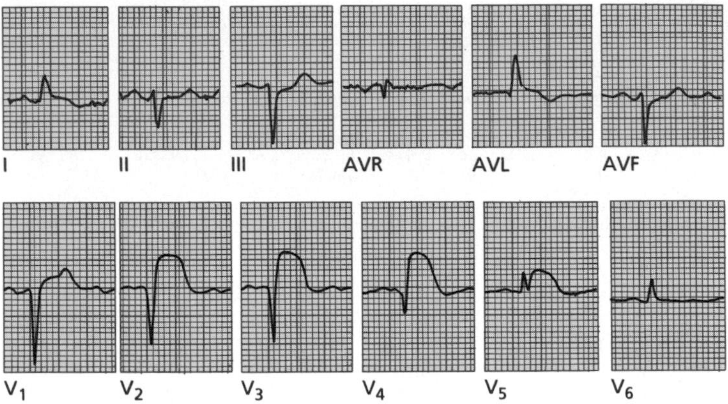

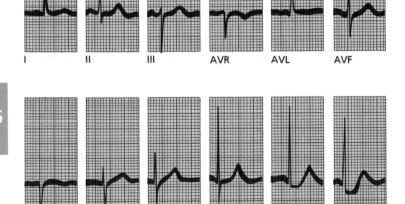

Fig. 5.23 Anterior myocardial infarction.

Fig. 5.24 Myocardial ischaemia (clinical history essential). The main characteristic is a depressed ST segment in leads standard II and V. Also not inverted U waves in II, III, AVF and V_{4-6}.

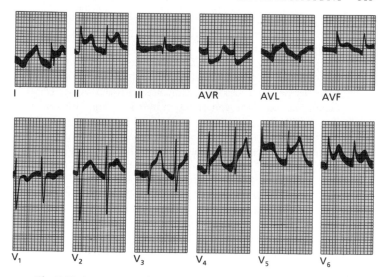

Fig. 5.25 Acute pericarditis. Raised concave-upwards ST segments in most leads, maximal in leads II and V$_{5-6}$.

Common abnormalities
Rhythm
Causes of bradycardia

Sinus (originating from sinoatrial (SA) node; normal P waves) — 'physiological' (e.g. athletes), beta-blockers, hypothyroidism, hypothermia.

Complete heart block.

Possible causes of tachycardia

Narrow complex tachycardia Normal duration of QRS complex, i.e. depolarization starts in or above the AV node.

Supraventricular tachycardia, atrial tachycardia If the rate of supraventricular depolarization is about 150/minute (one beat for every two large squares), the ventricles usually follow beat for beat. The P waves can sometimes be found in the preceding T wave.

If the atrial depolarization arises in or close to the AV node (*nodal* or *junctional tachycardia*), the P wave may be buried in the QRS complex.

If the rate of supraventricular depolarization is over 200/minute, AV block occurs and only some (2 : 1, or 3 : 1) episodes of atrial depolarization are followed by ventricular depolarization – the ventricles cannot keep up with the atria (Fig. 5.26).

At an atrial rate of 300/minute (one to every large square), there is a sawtooth baseline and the rhythm is called *atrial flutter* (Fig. 5.27). (The ventricular rate is then 150/minute in 2 : 1 block and 100/minute in 3 : 1 block.)

Atrial fibrillation (Fig. 5.28) Uncoordinated contraction of separate atrial muscle fibres. Unless 'controlled' by digoxin, it is usually fast (>120/minute), is totally irregular without P waves and has an irregular baseline.

Broad complex tachycardia Wide and abnormal QRS complex, i.e. depolarization starts above the AV node with abnormal

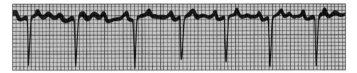

Fig. 5.26 Supraventricular tachycardia with varying AV block.

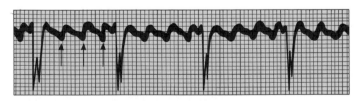

Fig. 5.27 Atrial flutter with 'sawtooth' atrial waves.

conduction below it (*supraventricular tachycardia with aberrant ventricular conduction*) or depolarization starts below the AV node (*ventricular tachycardia*).

Ventricular tachycardia (Fig. 5.29) P waves are absent or dissociated from QRS complexes; the QRS complexes vary in shape and are often very broad. It can be difficult to distinguish from supraventricular tachycardia with aberrant conduction. The diagnosis is favoured by the presence of a known cardiac abnormality (ischaemic heart disease or cardiomyopathy).

Ventricular fibrillation Very rapid irregular ventricular activation causes a sawtooth appearance (Fig. 5.30) — it is associated with no mechanical output, resulting in cardiac arrest (p. 306).

Occasional *extrasystoles* (ectopic or extra beats which do not

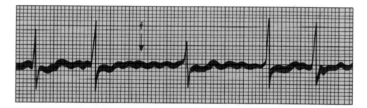

Fig. 5.28 Atrial fibrillation.

5

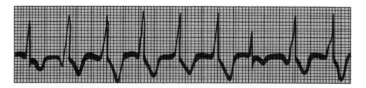

Fig. 5.29 Ventricular tachycardia with slightly irregular 'ventricular' QRS complexes and variable T waves due to dissociated superimposed P waves.

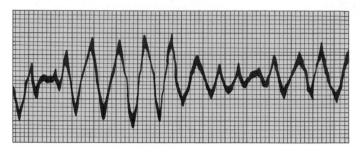

Fig. 5.30 Ventricular fibrillation. This is often seen in 'cardiac arrest' and may be irreversible. It may sometimes alternate with ventricular tachycardia (and sinus rhythm).

fit in the otherwise regular rhythm) occur normally. The QRS complex may be normal (atrial or supraventricular) (Fig. 5.31) or wide (ventricular or supraventricular with aberrant conduction; Fig. 5.32).

ECG patterns in common clinical conditions

Myocardial infarction A characteristic pattern of ECG changes evolves.

First few minutes — peaked T waves.

First few hours — ST segment elevation, inversion of T waves.

After the first few hours Q waves develop.

After a few days the ST segment returns to normal (persistent

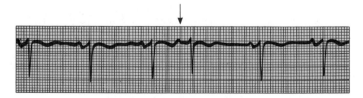

Fig. 5.31 Atrial extrasystole.

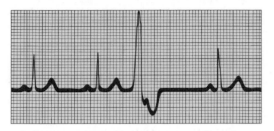

Fig. 5.32 Ventricular ectopic beat. A bizarre 'ventricular' QRS complex. These are more ominous if multifocal, i.e. QRS of varying shape.

elevation raises the possibility of LV aneurysm).

The T waves may eventually become upright but Q waves persist indefinitely.

Rhythm abnormalities are common.

Bundle branch block may occur at any stage, making further interpretation of the site, timing or extent of an infarct impossible.

Pulmonary embolism (Fig. 5.33)

Tachycardia and transient arrhythmias (particularly atrial fibrillation).

Right axis deviation.

RV strain pattern — dominant R wave and inverted T waves in V_1-V_4.

Right bundle branch block.

Occasionally S_1, Q_3, T_3 pattern (S wave in lead I, Q and inverted T in III).

Ventricular hypertrophy

Large R waves occur over the appropriate ventricle in the chest leads (V_1-V_2 for right and V_5-V_6 for left). There tend to be large negative S waves in reciprocal leads (e.g. large S in V_1 in LV hypertrophy). If the sum of the S in V_1 plus the R in V_5 is greater than 35 mm, LV hypertrophy is present on voltage criteria.

Digoxin Sagging (reverse tick) ST segments, T wave inversion.

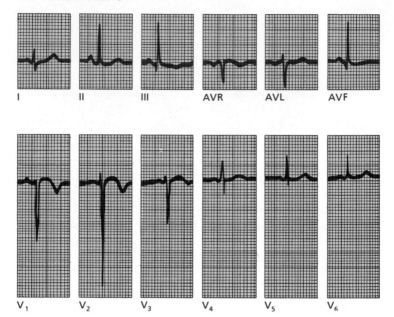

Fig. 5.33 Acute pulmonary embolism with S_1, Q_3, T_3 pattern, a mean frontal QRS axis towards the right (+90°) and 'RV strain' pattern in leads V_{1-3}.

Metabolic abnormalities

Hyperkalaemia (Fig. 5.34) — flattened P wave, broad QRS complex, peaked T wave.

Hypokalaemia (Fig. 5.34) — prolonged PR, depressed ST, flattened T wave and prominent U wave.

Hypocalcaemia (Fig. 5.35) — prolonged QT interval.

LUNG FUNCTION

Arterial blood gases

Give information about acid–base balance and about oxygen and carbon dioxide exchange and carriage.

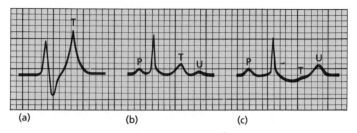

Fig. 5.34 (a) Hyperkalaemia, (b) normal and (c) hypokalaemia. The T wave amplitude varies directly with the serum potassium and the U wave inversely (it is often normally present in V_{3-4}). In hyperkalaemia the P waves become smaller and the QRS complex widens into the ST segment. In hypokalaemia the PR interval lengthens and the ST segment becomes depressed.

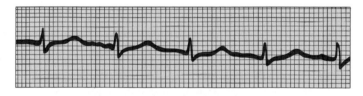

Fig. 5.35 Hypocalcaemia. Normal complexes apart from a prolonged QT_c (QT interval corrected for heart rate). (Rate 95/min, QT 0.40, QT_c 0.50.)

Reference values breathing air:

pH	7.36−7.44
partial pressure of arterial carbon dioxide (Pa_{CO_2})	4.7−6.0 kPa
partial pressure of arterial oxygen (Pa_{O_2})	10.7−13.3 kPa

Check the pH

If the pH is reduced, the patient has an acidosis; if raised an alkalosis.

Acidosis

If $PaCO_2$ is raised (hypercapnia), the acidosis is primarily respiratory.

If $PaCO_2$ is low, the acidosis is primarily metabolic.

Alkalosis

If $PaCO_2$ is low, the alkalosis is primarily respiratory.

If $PaCO_2$ is raised, the alkalosis is primarily metabolic.

Disorders which primarily affect entry of air into the alveoli (e.g. asthma) reduce the clearance of CO_2 from the lungs, and put up the $PaCO_2$.

Disorders which primarily affect exchange of gas within the alveoli (e.g. fibrosing alveolitis) usually lower the PaO_2 (hypoxia). The $PaCO_2$ is often normal or low as the patient may hyperventilate and CO_2 diffuses easily, so that defects in one part of the lungs can be readily compensated for in other parts. However, oxygen exchange when reduced in one part of the lungs cannot be compensated by good function in other parts.

Hypercapnia with a normal PaO_2 suggests that there is a modest reduction in ventilation (e.g. asthma).

Hypoxia without hypercapnia suggests a mismatch of ventilation and perfusion in a considerable part of the lungs (e.g. multiple pulmonary emboli, chronic bronchitis).

Ventilatory function tests

Peak expiratory flow rate (PEFR)

From maximal inspiration, with maximal but brief expiratory force, this is the flow over the first 10 milliseconds. It is reduced by airway narrowing, as in asthma and chronic bronchitis, or with respiratory muscle weakness. It is falsely low if the patient does not give maximum effort from maximum inhaled lung capacity, or if there is a leak at the mouthpiece. (Test your own to see how the peak flow meter is used and to gain some idea of PEFR in normal fit adults.)

Spirometry

From maximal inspiration and with maximal sustained expiratory force, the patient blows, usually into a dry wedge spirometer

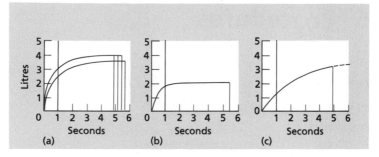

Fig. 5.36 Spirometric patterns. (a) Normal (elderly man): $FEV_1/FVC = 3.0/4.0 = 75\%$. (b) Restrictive: $FEV_1/FVC_i = 1.8/2.0 = 90\%$.
(c) Obstructive: $FEV_1/FVC = 1.4/3.5 = 40\%$.

(Vitalograph), as fast and completely as possible.

Forced expiratory volume (FEV_1) is the volume exhaled in the first second and forced vital capacity (FVC) the total volume exhaled overall (Fig. 5.36). The ratio of these two values may be expressed as a percentage, i.e. $(FEV_1/FVC) \times 100$.

FEV_1 and FVC are age, sex and height dependent (refer to charts for normal ranges).

$FEV_1/FVC\%$ is normally 70–80%.

Obstructive pattern (asthma, chronic bronchitis) In airflow obstruction, where FEV_1 is reduced more than FVC, the $FEV_1/FVC\%$ is usually reduced well below 60%.

Restrictive pattern (e.g. fibrosing alveolitis) In parenchymal lung disease, when the airways may be normal but the lungs restricted in movement, most and occasionally all the lung volume may be exhaled within the first second, giving an abnormally high $FEV_1/FVC\%$ with a much reduced FVC.

5

6 Procedures

6

INTRODUCTION

Practical procedures are best learnt by observing an experienced operator, and then performing the procedure under close supervision. Invasive procedures are frightening for patients, particularly if they have not experienced them before. Always explain carefully to the patient before the procedure what you are going to do, and what you expect from them.

TAKING BLOOD

Procedure

Ensure the patient is sitting or lying down.

Apply a tourniquet (or sphygmomanometer cuff inflated to about 40 mmHg — i.e. below diastolic blood pressure (BP)) around the upper arm.

Choose a vein — the cephalic, median cubital or basilic veins (Fig. 6.1) of the antecubital fossa are commonly used. It is easier to take blood from a vein that is easily palpable (and therefore distended with blood) than one that is readily visible, but less easy to feel.

Clean the skin with a swab (although this is considered by some to be unnecessary, it ensures that the skin is clean, often makes the veins more prominent, and ensures you have a swab available at the end of the procedure to compress the venepuncture site).

Prepare the needle (usually 21 gauge or green) and syringe Insert the needle in through the skin and into the vein — you should feel the needle give as it first enters the skin, and then as it enters the vein. Do not hesitate as you pierce the skin — the most pain is usually experienced as the needle enters or leaves the skin.

Hold the syringe with the left hand and withdraw the plunger with the right hand until the required amount of blood is collected.

Release the tourniquet.

Gently press the swab against the puncture site, and in one movement withdraw the needle from the vein and skin.

Press on the site until bleeding ceases (usually about 30 seconds).

6

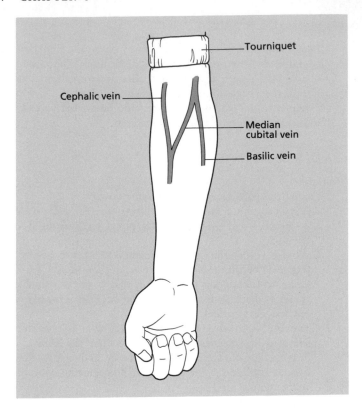

Fig. 6.1 Taking blood: the cephalic, basilic and median cubital veins.

Do not bend the arm as this increases the risk of bruising. Remove and discard the needle.

Do not resheathe the needle: the commonest cause of needle-stick injury.

Put the blood into correct bottles with appropriate anti-coagulant:

- plain tube (clotted sample) for serum;
- heparin for plasma;
- fluoride (stabilizes glucose by inhibiting glycolysis) for glucose;
- ethylenediamine tetra-acetic acid (EDTA) (prevents clotting by chelating calcium) for full blood count.

INSERTING AN INTRAVENOUS CANNULA

Indications

Administration of intravenous fluids or medication.

Procedure

The patient should be lying, with the arm to be cannulated by their side. It is a sensible precaution to put a disposable towel under the arm.

Apply a tourniquet or BP cuff around the upper arm. Choose a vein — the left (or right in left-handed people) forearm, away from the wrist and elbow, is the most convenient site. Shaving excess hair from the arm avoids discomfort for the patient when the cannula and surrounding tape are removed.

Clean the site with alcohol or iodine (ask about sensitivity if using iodine). Cannulae consist of a plastic sheath with a central metal needle (usually with a reservoir to collect blood at the end; Fig. 6.2).

Insert the needle and cannula through the skin and into the vein. Once the vein is entered the reservoir will start to fill with blood. Advance the needle a few millimetres further to ensure it is in the vein, withdraw the needle slightly and advance the plastic cannula over it until the hub is in contact with the skin.

Release the tourniquet.

Press over the tip of the cannula in the vein (to prevent blood flowing back through the cannula), withdraw the needle completely and either flush with saline and place a sterile cap on the cannula, or connect an intravenous infusion if required. Tape the cannula securely in place.

Complications

Failure to find or cannulate a vein Release the tourniquet; press over the site of any attempt, to prevent bruising. Do not despair — find a more experienced person. If no suitable veins are available, a 'cut-down' (exposing a vein through a small incision) may be necessary. Alternatively a central vein (subclavian or jugular) may be cannulated (see below).

Inflammation Due to infection or thrombophlebitis.

Remove the cannula and resite a new one. Inflammation

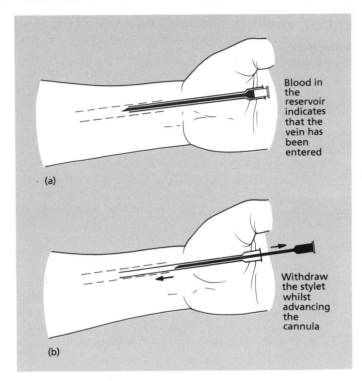

Fig. 6.2 Peripheral vein cannulation.

usually settles once the cannula is removed.

Blockage Usually due to clotting of the cannula or vein, or the cannula slipping out of the vein.

Remove and resite.

CENTRAL VEIN CANNULATION

Several approaches for cannulation of central veins are available. All are potentially hazardous, and should only be performed by, or under the close supervision of, an experienced operator. The infraclavicular approach to subclavian vein cannulation will be described here.

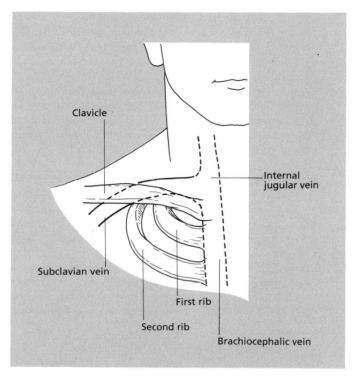

Fig. 6.3 Subclavian vein: anatomy.

Anatomy (Fig. 6.3)

The subclavian vein is a continuation of the axillary vein. It begins at the outer border of the first rib, which it arches over, and passes medially to join the internal jugular vein and form the brachiocephalic vein.

Procedure

The patient should lie flat without pillows. Tilting the bed 5–10° head down helps to fill the vein. Either side may be used, although the right is more common. The head is turned to the opposite side.

Sterility should be maintained at all times — wear a mask, gown and gloves, clean a wide area around the mid-point of the clavicle, and cover the surrounding area with sterile towels.

Identify the mid-point of the clavicle and infiltrate the skin below the lower border of the bone with local anaesthetic (e.g. 1% lignocaine).

Attach a syringe to the cannula, which is usually a longer version of a peripheral intravenous cannula, and insert the needle below the mid-point of the clavicle (Fig. 6.4). Slowly advance the needle beneath the clavicle, aiming at the supra-sternal notch. Whilst advancing the needle, gently aspirate on the syringe — dark (venous) blood will flush back as the vein is entered.

Advance the needle and cannula a few millimetres further to ensure it is in the vein, withdraw the needle slightly, and slide the cannula over the needle into the vein. The needle is then withdrawn, and the cannula sealed with a bung or syringe or by connecting an infusion, to prevent aspiration of air into the central vein.

The cannula is then usually replaced by a central venous catheter using the *Seldinger technique* (Fig. 6.5). After introducing the cannula, a flexible guide wire is passed through the cannula into the vessel and the cannula removed, leaving just the guide

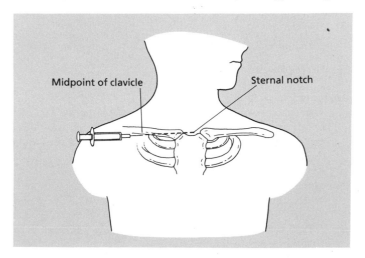

Fig. 6.4 Insertion of cannula for subclavian vein catheterization.

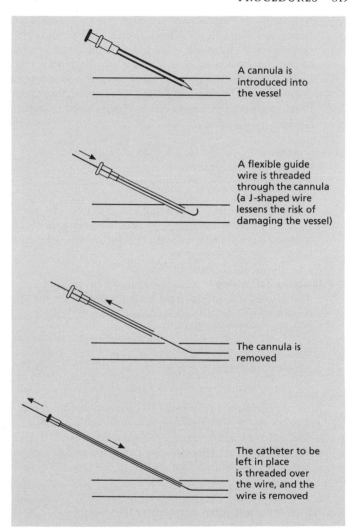

A cannula is introduced into the vessel

A flexible guide wire is threaded through the cannula (a J-shaped wire lessens the risk of damaging the vessel)

The cannula is removed

The catheter to be left in place is threaded over the wire, and the wire is removed

6

Fig. 6.5 Seldinger technique.

wire in place. The catheter to be left *in situ* (which is usually longer and more flexible than the original cannula) is then threaded over the guide wire, and the guide wire removed.

The catheter is then secured in place, usually with a suture.

A chest X-ray should always be taken to ensure correct positioning of the catheter (the tip should be in the right atrium), and check that a pneumothorax has not been caused by puncturing the apex of the lung.

Complications

Injury to thoracic structures

- Pneumothorax;
- haemothorax;
- arterial puncture — bright red blood (unless the patient is hypoxic) pulsates from the cannula. The cannula should be removed immediately, and direct pressure applied to the site for at least 10 minutes;
- injury to the thoracic duct.

Infection Strict aseptic technique should be maintained at the time of insertion, and at all subsequent times when the catheter is used.

Subclavian vein thrombosis

ARTERIAL PUNCTURE

Indications

Arterial puncture is performed to measure arterial blood gases and pH.

The radial or brachial artery is usually punctured — the femoral artery may also be used, although this site is less convenient and the artery is in close proximity to the larger femoral vein.

Radial artery puncture: procedure

The patient should be sitting or lying.

Choose a site about 1 cm proximal to the wrist joint where the artery can be readily felt.

Raise a small bleb of local anaesthetic in the overlying skin with an orange (25 gauge) needle.

Draw up less than 0.5 ml of 1000 U/ml heparin into a 2 ml syringe through a blue (23 gauge) needle, and squirt most of it away to leave a small amount in the tip. Ensure there is no air in the syringe.

Palpate the radial artery with the index finger of the left hand. With the right hand insert the needle, attached to the heparinized syringe, through the skin at an angle of 45°. Slowly advance the needle towards the pulse until arterial blood pulses into the syringe. Collect the necessary amount of blood (usually about 2 ml).

Remove the needle and apply firm pressure over the puncture site for 5 minutes.

The needle should be removed and the syringe capped. The sample is then taken for immediate analysis. If there is likely to be any delay in analysing the sample it should be cooled in ice, and subsequently rewarmed to body temperature.

Complications

Haematoma.

Arterial thrombosis or embolism.

Aneurysm formation.

Arteriovenous fistula formation.

PLEURAL ASPIRATION

Indications

Diagnosis

Aspiration of fluid to look for pus (empyema) or blood (haemothorax).

Microscopy and culture to look for infection.

Cytology for malignant cells.

Protein estimation (to distinguish transudate from exudate — p. 335).

Treatment

Drainage of blood or pus.

Removal of fluid to relieve dyspnoea.

Procedure

The patient should sit, leaning slightly forward, with their arms

6

placed over a rest (e.g. a bed table or the back of a chair).

Locate the site for aspiration by percussion and comparison with X-rays. The usual site is posteriorly in the mid-line.

Wear a mask and gloves and clean a wide area around the site.

Infiltrate local anaesthetic (e.g. 1% lignocaine) into the skin in the lower part of the intercostal space (to avoid the neurovascular bundle on the undersurface of each rib) with an orange (25 gauge) needle. With a green needle infiltrate down to and through the pleura until fluid can be withdrawn.

If the tap is only for diagnosis, 20–50 ml of fluid are aspirated into a sterile syringe.

To remove larger quantities of fluid a needle attached to a three-way tap is used — fluid is aspirated into the syringe, the tap is switched, and the fluid drained via a tube into a sterile container. When removing large volumes of fluid it is often easier, and more comfortable for the patient, to introduce a catheter, such as an intravenous cannula, remove the stylet and attach the three-way tap to the catheter.

PLEURAL BIOPSY

Pleural biopsy should be performed at the same time as pleural aspiration if the cause of the effusion is not known. The Abrams' needle (Fig. 6.6), consisting of an inner and an outer trocar with a biopsy port, and an inner stylet, is most commonly used.

Procedure

The patient is positioned, and the site prepared and anaesthetized, as for pleural aspiration.

Make a small incision through the skin and into the intercostal muscle with a no. 11 scalpel blade.

Insert the biopsy needle into the pleural cavity (Fig. 6.7).

Withdraw the inner trocar to expose the biopsy port.

Slowly withdraw the trocar until it is felt to catch on the pleura.

Take a sample of pleura by turning the stylet to close the biopsy port.

Withdraw the whole needle.

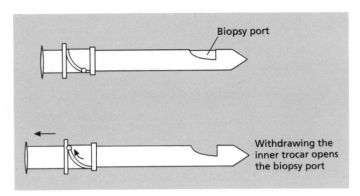

Fig. 6.6 Abrams' needle.

RECORDING AN ELECTROCARDIOGRAM (ECG)

Procedure

The patient should lie down and relax.

Calibrate the ECG machine — a standard signal of 1 mV should move the stylus two large squares (1 cm) vertically.

Attach the limb leads: left arm (LA); right arm (RA); left leg (LL); right leg (RL).

Record the six standard leads (I, II, III, augmented voltage right arm (AVR), augmented voltage left arm (AVL), augmented voltage foot (AVF)) by turning the dial on the ECG machine — three or four complexes for each.

Apply the electrode to the six chest positions in turn (Fig. 6.8), recording three to four complexes of each.

- V_1 — fourth right intercostal space, parasternal;
- V_2 — fourth left intercostal space, parasternal;
- V_3 — fourth/fifth left intercostal space, between sternum and mid-clavicular line;
- V_4 — fifth left intercostal space, mid-clavicular line;
- V_5 — fifth left intercostal space, anterior axillary line;
- V_6 — fifth left intercostal space, mid-axillary line.

If the rhythm does not appear to be sinus, a rhythm strip of 6–10 complexes in a single lead should be recorded.

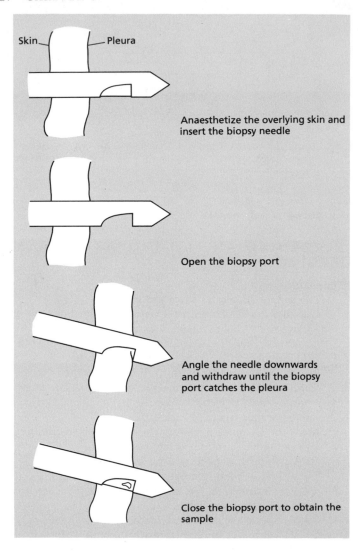

Skin — Pleura

Anaesthetize the overlying skin and insert the biopsy needle

Open the biopsy port

Angle the needle downwards and withdraw until the biopsy port catches the pleura

Close the biopsy port to obtain the sample

Fig. 6.7 Pleural biopsy.

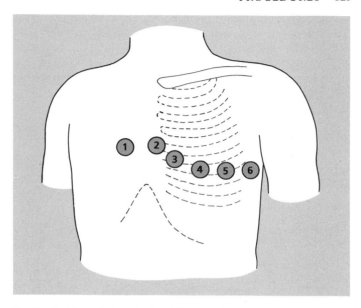

Fig. 6.8 Position of chest leads whilst recording an ECG.

PASSING A NASOGASTRIC TUBE

Indications

Aspiration of stomach contents.

Maintenance of nutrition in patients who are unable to swallow.

Procedure

The patient should be sitting comfortably.

Select a tube — for gastric aspiration a large rigid tube (e.g. 16 French gauge), which is unlikely to block, is preferred, whereas a fine-bore tube with a wire introducer may be used for feeding.

Lubricate the tip of the tube with KY jelly.

Slide the tube into the nostril until you feel it hit the nasopharynx.

Ask the patient to swallow (give them a glass of water if not contraindicated) and continue to advance the tube down into the oesophagus.

6

Continue to advance the tube into the stomach (Fig. 6.9).

Several methods help in signifying when the tube is in the
stomach:

  • tubes usually have three marks which indicate roughly
  when the tube should reach the oesophagogastric junction,
  antrum and pylorus;

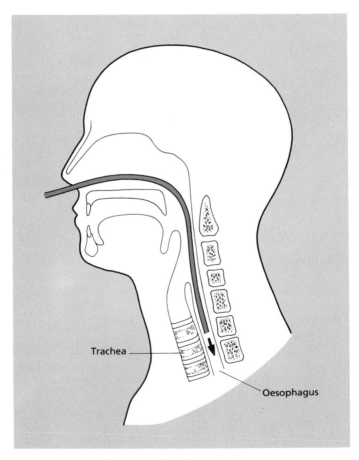

Fig. 6.9 Insertion of a nasogastric tube.

- if the tube is in the stomach, air blown down the tube with a syringe may be heard entering the stomach by listening with a stethoscope over the upper left quadrant;
- aspirate the tube for gastric contents — the presence of acid (test with litmus paper) indicates that the tube is in the stomach.

If there is doubt about the position of the tube it may be checked by X-ray.

Once in the correct position the tube should be secured firmly to the nose with tape.

Complications

Tracheal intubation — choking usually indicates that the tube is in the trachea and should be withdrawn immediately.

Obstruction of the tube due to blockage or twisting.

Nasal or oesophageal erosions.

PARACENTESIS (TAPPING ABDOMINAL FLUID)

Indications

Small volumes (up to 50 ml) of abdominal fluid are usually removed for diagnostic purposes — to measure protein content (to distinguish transudate from exudate — p. 340) or amylase or to look for malignant cells or infection.

Drainage of large volumes to relieve discomfort is usually precluded by the risk of hypovolaemia, but may be necessary in patients with intra-abdominal malignancy.

Procedure

Confirm the presence of ascites (pp. 100−1).

The patient should empty their bladder and then lie comfortably on their back.

Select a site for paracentesis — usually an area in one of the iliac fossae where there is shifting dullness (away from solid organs — the location of the liver and spleen should be confirmed by palpation and percussion).

Wear a mask and gloves and clean a wide area around the site.

Infiltrate the skin and down to the parietal peritoneum with local anaesthetic (e.g. 1% lignocaine).

6

Attach a long, fine needle (e.g. 23 gauge) to a 50 ml syringe and introduce the needle through the skin and fascia into the abdominal cavity. Aspirate gently as the needle is advanced — fluid will flow back once the needle is in the correct place.

Send fluid to the laboratory for cell count and differential, cytology, culture, protein concentration and, if pancreatitis is suspected, enzyme estimation.

For drainage of larger volumes of fluid a plastic cannula is usually introduced into the abdominal cavity and fluid drained into a sterile closed drainage system.

Complications

Inadvertent puncture of the intestine is unusual, and rarely leads to complications.

URETHRAL CATHETERIZATION

Indications

Relief of urinary retention (e.g. due to prostatic hypertrophy or neurogenic bladder).

Prevention of urinary incontinence due to debility.

To obtain a urine specimen or measure residual urine.

To introduce contrast media prior to radiography of the urinary tract.

Procedure

Unless drainage of a considerable amount of blood or debris is anticipated, a small, soft catheter (e.g. 12–14 French gauge) should be used to minimize trauma to the urethra.

Wear a mask and gloves and adopt a strict aseptic technique.

Men

The patient should lie comfortably on his back.

Retract the prepuce and thoroughly clean the glans and meatus with 0.5% chlorhexidine.

Place sterile towels around the penis, which itself can be wrapped in gauze.

Introduce 1% lignocaine jelly into the urethra using a plastic nozzle.

Allow about 5 minutes for the jelly to anaesthetize the urethra.

Gently slide the catheter through the meatus into the urethra, with the free end in a sterile receiver. A small amount of resistance (due to involuntary muscle spasm) is usually encountered as the catheter meets the external sphincter. The catheter is then advanced into the bladder and urine flows back into the receiver. Occasionally the tube may become blocked by jelly and gentle aspiration is required to establish a flow of urine.

Insert the catheter as far as possible into the bladder (to ensure it is not in the urethra), inflate the balloon with the appropriate volume of sterile water, and then withdraw the catheter until resistance is felt as the balloon rests against the bladder neck.

Connect the catheter to a sterile closed drainage system.

Women

The procedure in women is much simpler as the female urethra is only 2–3 cm long.

The patient should lie on her back with her knees flexed and thighs abducted.

Clean the labia and surrounding skin with chlorhexidine, and place sterile towels around the surrounding area.

Part the labia majoris and minoris and identify the urethral meatus beneath the clitoris.

Lubricate the catheter with KY jelly and gently insert it through the meatus into the bladder until urine flows.

Inflate the balloon and connect the catheter to a sterile closed drainage system.

Complications

Infection.

Urethral stricture formation.

Traumatic catheterization with urethral rupture.

6

LUMBAR PUNCTURE

Indications

Diagnosis of:
* meningitis;

- subarachnoid haemorrhage (cranial computed tomography (CT) scanning usually yields more information and is less hazardous or traumatic to the patient);
- inflammatory disorders (e.g. multiple sclerosis, Guillain–Barré).

Introducing contrast media (myelography).

Introducing chemotherapeutic agents (e.g. in leukaemia).

Contraindications

Raised intracranial pressure.

Coagulation defects (subdural, epidural or intrathecal haematomas may compress the cord).

Procedure

The patient should lie on their left side with their back right up against the edge of the bed, and their knees drawn up to their chin. Ensure that the back is at 90° to the bed by positioning the shoulders and pelvis vertically.

Identify and draw a line between the anterior superior iliac spines. This lies at the level of the L3–L4 interspace, which can be used to perform the lumbar puncture (Fig. 6.10). In

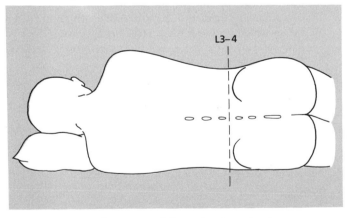

Fig. 6.10 Position of a patient whilst performing a lumbar puncture.

adults the spinal cord ends at L1–L2, so the L2–L3 or L4–L5 space is also acceptable.

Strict aseptic technique should be maintained throughout the procedure — wear a mask, gown and gloves, clean a wide area around the lumbar spine, and cover the surrounding area with sterile towels.

Palpate the spinous processes above and below the chosen inter-space and infiltrate the skin and deeper tissues with local anaesthetic (e.g. 1% lignocaine).

Introduce the spinal needle (an outer metal sheath with an inner metal stylet) between the spinous processes, at right angles to the back, aiming towards the umbilicus.

Push the needle through the resistance of the superficial supra-spinous ligament and across the interspinous ligament. The resistance of the ligamentum flavum is then encountered — the needle will be felt to 'give' as this is crossed and the subarachnoid space entered (Fig. 6.11).

The stylet is then withdrawn, and cerebrospinal fluid (CSF) should drip out.

Once flow of fluid is obtained, attach a manometer via a three-way tap and measure the CSF pressure (normal 80–180 mm), which should rise and fall freely with respiration.

If a greatly raised CSF pressure (over 250 mm) is recorded, the fluid from the manometer should be collected and the needle withdrawn.

Collect three or four drops of CSF into three sterile containers (labelled in order of collection) for cell count and differential, protein estimation, culture and serology. If meningitis is suspected collect a few drops into a fluoride tube for glucose estimation (see pp. 266–7). If blood-stained CSF is obtained, further serial samples may be taken to determine whether the CSF clears with time, indicating a traumatic tap.

Once the fluid is collected, remove the needle and apply a plaster. The patient should be nursed flat for 24 hours.

Complications

Headache.

Haematoma.

Herniation of the brain through the foramen magnum ('coning')

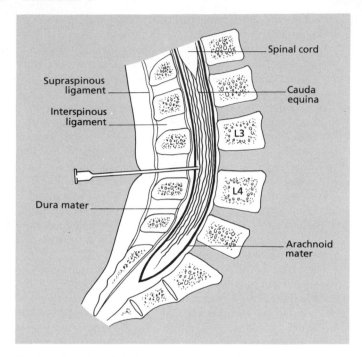

Fig. 6.11 Insertion of the lumbar puncture needle.

occurs when raised intracranial pressure is rapidly decompressed by the lumbar puncture. The process is rapidly fatal, and lumbar puncture should always be avoided if there is any suspicion of raised intracranial pressure.

6

7 Lists

7

LISTS OF COMMON MEDICAL CONDITIONS

(Included in text but consolidated for convenience.)

Causes

Clubbing

Pulmonary — malignancy (carcinoma, mesothelioma), chronic suppurative disease (abscess, empyema, bronchiectasis, cystic fibrosis, tuberculosis) and fibrosing alveolitis.

Cardiac — cyanotic heart disease and infective endocarditis.

Abdominal — inflammatory bowel disease, coeliac disease, cirrhosis.

Thyrotoxicosis (thyroid acropachy).

Congenital.

Lymphadenopathy

Localized

Local infection (including tuberculous).

Metastatic carcinoma.

Lymphoma (Hodgkin's and non-Hodgkin's).

Generalized

Infection (e.g. infectious mononucleosis, cytomegalovirus (CMV), *Toxoplasma*, rubella, human immunodeficiency virus (HIV).

Reticuloendothelial disorders.

Chronic lymphatic leukaemia.

Rare causes These include: sarcoidosis, connective tissue diseases (e.g. rheumatoid arthritis), drugs (e.g. phenytoin).

Haemoptysis

Infection (pneumonia, lung abscess).

Bronchial carcinoma.

Pulmonary embolism.

Pulmonary oedema (frothy blood-stained sputum).

Pulmonary tuberculosis.

Pulmonary vasculitis.

Foreign body.

Mitral stenosis (with pulmonary hypertension).
Coagulation disorders.

Large pleural effusion
Transudates (protein content less than 30 g/litre)
  Heart failure.
  Hypoproteinaemia (e.g. nephrotic syndrome, liver failure).
  Hypothyroidism (rare).
Exudates (protein content greater than 30 g/litre)
  Pneumonia.
  Malignancy (bronchial carcinoma, metastatic carcinoma, mesothelioma, lymphoma).
  Pulmonary infarction.
  Tuberculosis.
  Connective tissue disease.
  Subphrenic abscess.

Pneumothorax
Spontaneous
No underlying lung disease (usually young adult males).
Secondary to underlying lung disease:
- localized or diffuse bullae;
- asthma;
- tuberculosis;
- lung abscess;
- malignancy.

Traumatic
Iatrogenic (e.g. following thoracic surgery, artificial ventilation)

Hypertension
Essential (95%).
Alcohol.
Coarctation of the aorta.
Renal disease.
Endocrine disease:
- Cushing's (increased adrenal corticosteroids);
- Conn's syndrome (increased adrenal mineralocorticoids);
- phaeochromocytoma (increased adrenaline and noradrenaline from adrenal medulla);

7

- acromegaly;
- contraceptive pill;
- eclampsia (toxaemia) of pregnancy.

Atrial fibrillation
Cardiac
Ischaemic heart disease.
Hypertension.
Cardiomyopathy.
Rheumatic valve disease.
Atrial septal defect.
Pericarditis.
Atrial myxoma.
Pulmonary
Pulmonary embolus.
Cor pulmonale.
Bronchial carcinoma.
Thyrotoxicosis

Left-sided heart failure
Hypertension.
Myocardial ischaemia.
Mitral and aortic valve disease.
Cardiomyopathy.
Cardiac arrythmia.
Viral myocarditis.

Right-sided heart failure
Secondary to left-sided heart failure
Pulmonary hypertension due to
Chronic obstructive airways disease (cor pulmonale).
Mitral valve stenosis.
Recurrent pulmonary emboli.
Left-to-right cardiac shunts.
Pulmonary stenosis.

Raised jugular venous pulse (JVP)
Non-pulsatile
Superior mediastinal compression.

Platysmal compression.
Large goitre (rare).
Pulsatile
Heart failure.
Airways obstruction (asthma, bronchitis).
Fluid overload.
Cardiac tamponade (rare).

Large 'a' wave
Pulmonary hypertension.
Pulmonary stenosis.
Tricuspid stenosis.

Cannon wave (giant 'a' wave)
Regular — nodal rhythm.
Irregular — complete heart block.

Absent 'a' wave
Atrial fibrillation.

Large 'v' wave
Tricuspid regurgitation (confirm by palpation of pulsatile liver).

Aortic stenosis
Valvar stenosis
Congenital
- True congenital aortic stenosis;
- calcification of a bicuspid valve.

Acquired
- Rheumatic fever.

Subvalvar stenosis
Congenital.
Hypertrophic obstructive cardiomyopathy.

Supravalvar aortic stenosis
Congenital, often associated with abnormal facies.

Aortic regurgitation
Valve abnormality
Rheumatic fever.

7

Congenital: bicuspid or deficient valve.

Infective endocarditis (usually on an abnormal valve).

Aortic root dilatation

Hypertension.

Aortic dissection.

Ankylosing spondylitis.

Reiter's syndrome.

Marfan's syndrome.

Syphilis.

Mitral regurgitation

Floppy (prolapsing) mitral valve leaflets.

Ischaemic papillary muscle dysfunction, particularly after inferior myocardial infarction.

Left ventricular failure with dilatation of mitral valve ring.

Rheumatic fever.

Cardiomyopathy.

Mitral stenosis

Rheumatic fever.

Very rarely congenital.

Haematemesis

Gastric erosion.

Oesophagitis and Mallory—Weiss tears (i.e. tears of the oesophageal mucosa after forceful vomiting).

Duodenal ulcer.

Gastric ulcer (benign or malignant).

Oesophageal varices (dilated oesophageal veins due to portal venous hypertension).

Coagulation disorders.

Hepatomegaly

Common causes

Cardiac failure.

Secondary carcinomatous deposits.

Cirrhosis.

Other causes

Infection — viral (hepatitis, glandular fever), bacterial (liver abscess) or parasitic (amoebic abscess, hydatid cysts).

Reticuloendothelial disorders (leukaemia, myelofibrosis, lymphoma).

Amyloidosis.

Sarcoidosis.

Storage disease (glycogen, lipid).

Primary hepatoma.

Haemochromatosis.

Primary biliary cirrhosis.

Wilson's disease.

Hepatic vein thrombosis (Budd—Chiari syndrome).

Polycystic disease.

Riedel's lobe (normal anatomical variant with enlargement of the right lobe).

Splenomegaly

Common causes of massive splenomegaly

Chronic myeloid leukaemia.

Myelofibrosis.

Malaria and kala-azar (visceral leishmaniasis).

Common causes of moderate splenomegaly

Reticuloendothelial disease.

Liver disease with portal hypertension (cirrhosis, Budd—Chiari).

Common causes of mild splenomegaly — infections

Glandular fever.

Hepatitis.

Brucellosis.

Infective endocarditis.

Rare causes of splenomegaly

Amyloidosis — deposition of immunoglobin or acute phase proteins in tissues in association with paraproteinaemia, chronic inflammation or chronic sepsis.

Sarcoidosis.

Storage diseases.

7

Connective tissue diseases.

Splenic abscess.

Hepatosplenomegaly

Infective (e.g. glandular fever, hepatitis).

Myeloproliferative disorders (e.g. myelofibrosis, chronic myeloid leukaemia).

Liver disease with portal hypertension.

Reticuloendothelial disease.

Storage diseases.

Cirrhosis

Common

Alcohol.

Cryptogenic (cause unknown).

Chronic active hepatitis — following hepatitis B or C; autoimmune.

Primary biliary cirrhosis (autoimmune).

Rarer causes

Secondary biliary cirrhosis (e.g. biliary stricture).

Budd–Chiari syndrome.

Metabolic:

- Haemochromatosis (iron deposition);
- Wilson's disease (copper deposition).

Enzyme deficiencies:

- α_1-Antitrypsin deficiency;
- galactosaemia;
- fructosaemia.

Glycogen storage disease.

Drugs (e.g. methotrexate).

Cystic fibrosis.

Chronic hepatic venous congestion (cardiac cirrhosis).

Ascites

Transudates (protein less than 30 g/litre)

Cirrhosis.

Hypoproteinaemia (e.g. nephrotic syndrome).

Exudate (protein greater than 30 g/litre)

Malignancy.

Infection (peritonitis, tuberculosis).

Pancreatitis.

Hepatic vein obstruction (Budd–Chiari syndrome).

Constrictive pericarditis.

Chylous Obstruction of main lymphatic duct (e.g. by carcinoma).

Dementia

Alzheimer's disease.

Multi-infarct dementia.

Subdural haematoma.

Malignancy (primary cerebral tumour or secondary).

Hypothyroidism (myxoedema madness).

Overmedication (particularly with sedatives).

Vitamin B_{12} deficiency.

Multiple sclerosis.

Acquired immunodeficiency syndrome (AIDS).

Huntington's chorea (autosomal dominant, gradual onset of dementia and ataxia in middle age).

Papilloedema

Raised intracranial pressure:
- cerebral tumour;
- cerebral abscess;
- meningitis;
- benign intracranial hypertension (young obese women with no intracranial lesion).

Malignant hypertension.

Retinal vein obstruction (central retinal vein thrombosis, cavernous sinus thrombosis).

Optic neuritis (inflammation of the optic nerve, most commonly due to multiple sclerosis).

Rarely metabolic causes (carbon dioxide (CO_2) retention in respiratory failure, hypoparathyroidism).

Peripheral neuropathy

Idiopathic.

Metabolic:
- diabetes mellitus;
- chronic renal failure;
- amyloidosis;

7

- acute intermittent porphyria.

Drugs (e.g. isoniazid, vincristine).

Heavy metals — lead, mercury.

Infection — tetanus, leprosy, diphtheria.

Vitamin deficiency B_{12} (subacute combined degeneration), B_1 (beriberi).

Connective tissue disease.

Sarcoidosis.

Guillain–Barré.

Malignancy.

Familial:

- hereditary ataxias;
- peroneal muscular atrophy.

Acute confusional states

Small strokes.

All of the system failures (cardiac, respiratory, hepatic, renal).

Severe acute infections, particularly with high fever (e.g. meningitis, pneumonia, malaria).

Drug overdose (e.g. alcohol, sedatives, salicylates, antidepressants).

Alcohol withdrawal.

Hypoglycaemia and hyperglycaemia.

Hypercalcaemia.

Endocrine disorders (e.g. thyrotoxicosis, hypothyroidism, Cushing's syndrome).

Proximal myopathy

Hypokalaemia.

Corticosteroid treatment and Cushing's syndrome.

Thyroid disease.

Acromegaly.

Alcoholism.

Osteomalacia.

Polymyositis.

Drugs (e.g. alcohol, lithium, chloroquine).

Muscular dystrophy.

Wasting of small muscles of hand

Old age; cachexia.

7

Rheumatoid arthritis.

Bilateral cervical ribs (compress T1).

Motor neurone disease.

Syringomyelia (cystic dilatation of central canal in cervical spinal cord).

Bilateral median and ulnar nerve lesions.

Signs

Large pleural effusion

Trachea usually central — deviated away from effusion if very large.

Diminished movement on side of effusion.

Over effusion: stony dull to percussion; diminished breath sounds (may be bronchial at top of effusion); diminished tactile vocal fremitus and vocal resonance.

Consolidation of lung

Trachea usually central — may be deviated towards lesion if associated collapse (collapse and consolidation often occur together).

Diminished movement on side of consolidation.

Over consolidation: dull to percussion; bronchial breathing; increased tactile vocal fremitus and vocal resonance (bronchial breathing absent with reduced tactile vocal fremitus and vocal resonance if airway obstructed, e.g. by carcinoma).

Lung collapse

Trachea deviated to side of collapse.

Diminished movement on side of collapse.

Over collapse: dull to percussion; diminished breath sound; diminished tactile vocal fremitus and vocal resonance (may be bronchial breathing with increased tactile vocal fremitus and vocal resonance).

Pneumothorax

Trachea usually central — may be deviated away if large.

Diminished movement on side of pneumothorax.

Percussion usually normal (hyperresonance may be detected).

7

Breath sounds, tactile vocal fremitus, vocal resonance are all diminished on side of pneumothorax.

Left-sided heart failure

Sinus (regular) tachycardia.

Hypotension.

Displacement of apex if there is hypertrophy or dilatation of the failing left ventricle.

Cardiac triple rhythm (third and/or fourth sound).

Fine bilateral basal crackles at lung bases posteriorly.

Signs of underlying cause (e.g. valve lesion).

Right-sided heart failure

Raised JVP.

Ankle and/or sacral oedema.

Liver enlargement and tenderness.

Signs of underlying cause.

Aortic stenosis

Plateau pulse.

Heaving apex.

Loud, harsh mid-systolic ejection murmur, best heard in second left intercostal space, radiating to carotids.

May be systolic ejection click.

Aortic regurgitation

Large-volume collapsing pulse (may be visible pulsation of carotids — Corrigan's sign).

Wide pulse pressure.

Apex displaced and heaving.

Blowing, high-pitched early diastolic murmur, loudest in third and fourth left intercostal space with patient sitting forward and breath held on expiration.

Mitral stenosis

Atrial fibrillation common, small-volume pulse (due to reduced cardiac output).

'Palpable' first sound.

Loud first sound on auscultation (unless valve mobility reduced by calcification).

7

Opening snap.

Mid-diastolic murmur — long, low frequency, rumbling murmur, best heard at the apex with patient rolled to left side.

Mitral regurgitation

Usually sinus rhythm (atrial fibrillation may occur).

Apex diffuse and thrusting, displaced laterally.

Apical pansystolic murmur radiating to the axilla.

Tricuspid regurgitation

Invariably atrial fibrillation.

Raised JVP with prominent systolic wave.

Prominent right ventricular impulse ('heave') at left sternal edge.

Pansystolic murmur *may* be heard at lower left sternal edge, loudest on inspiration.

Pulsatile, enlarged liver.

Ascites.

Oedema.

Ventricular septal defect (VSD)

Signs vary: small defect ('maladie de Roger') may give rise to loud murmur; but no other abnormal cardiovascular findings — large defect may cause pulmonary hypertension without a murmur.

Forceful apex and left parasternal heave if right ventricular hypertrophy.

Pansystolic murmur and thrill, maximal at lower left sternal edge.

Mid-diastolic mitral murmur if shunt is large.

Patent ductus arteriosus

Collapsing pulse.

Prominent apex (left ventricular hypertrophy).

Continuous 'machinery' murmur maximal under left clavicle.

Fallot's tetralogy

VSD.

Pulmonary stenosis.

Right ventricular hypertrophy.

'Overriding' aorta (the aorta is positioned over the VSD).

7

Cyanosis, clubbing, left parasternal heave of right ventricular hypertrophy, ejection systolic murmur of pulmonary stenosis (no murmur from large VSD).

Pulmonary hypertension

Malar flush — cyanosis or dusky pink discoloration of upper cheeks.

Small-volume pulse.

Atrial fibrillation.

Raised JVP — tricuspid regurgitation may be present.

Right parasternal heave (right ventricular hypertrophy).

'Palpable' pulmonary component of the second heart sound.

Enlarged liver — pulsatile if tricuspid regurgitation.

Ascites and peripheral oedema.

Ascites

Abdominal distension.

Dullness to percussion in flanks.

Shifting dullness.

Fluid thrill.

Peritonitis

Localized

Rebound tenderness.

Guarding.

Generalized

Shock: pale, cold skin, sweating, tachycardia, hypotension.

'Board-like' abdominal rigidity.

Absent bowel sounds.

Parkinson's disease

Triad of rigidity, tremor, bradykinesia (slow movement).

Signs

Flat affect and expressionless face.

Difficulty initiating movement (akinesia).

Rigid limbs — shuffling gait, and arms do not swing with walking.

Speech slurred and monotonous.

Tremor — pill rolling.

Cogwheel (due to superimposed tremor) rigidity of muscles —
best felt on moving wrists.

Depression.

Bulbar palsy

(Lower motor neurone palsy of cranial nerves IX, X, XII supplying
palatal, pharyngeal and tongue muscles.)

Nasal dysarthria.

Flaccid fasciculating tongue.

Normal or absent jaw jerk.

Pseudobulbar palsy

(Upper motor neurone palsy of cranial nerves IX, X, XII.)

Emotional lability.

'Donald Duck' speech.

Spastic tongue — small for mouth.

Increased jaw jerk.

Lower motor neurone lesion

Reduced or absent power.

Flaccid muscle wasting.

Absent reflexes and plantar response.

Upper motor neurone lesion

Reduced or absent power.

Increased muscle tone.

Exaggerated reflexes with clonus.

Upgoing plantars.

Cerebellar lesion

Signs on same side as lesion.

Incoordination, demonstrated by:

• dysdiadochokinesia;

• ataxic gait: reeling, staggering, tending to fall to side of
lesion.

Intention tremor.

Nystagmus: horizontal, more marked on looking to side of
lesion.

Dysarthria: slurred, explosive.

Horner's syndrome

Enophthalmos (the eyeball is indrawn).

Meiosis (small pupil).

Ptosis (drooping of the upper lid).

Anhydrosis (decreased sweating over the affected side of the face).

Index

Page numbers in *italics* refer to figures and tables.